LANCHESTER LIBRARY

3 8001 00512 2977

S

H

in

LANCHESTER LIBRARY, Coventry University
Gosford Street, Coventry CV1 ___ KT-472-265

ONE WEEK LOAN COLLECTION

CANCELLED 5 July (2nd)
CANCELLED 2 July (UK)
CANCELLED

19 JUL 2007

27 FEB 2007

18 APR 2007

CANCELLED

27 JUN 2007

This book is due to be returned not later than the date and
time stamped above. Fines are charged on overdue books

Published by the Remedica Group

Remedica Publishing Ltd, 32–38 Osnaburgh Street, London, NW1 3ND, UK
Remedica Inc, Tri-State International Center, Building 25, Suite 150, Lincolnshire, IL 60069, USA

E-mail: books@remedica.com
www.remedica.com

Publisher: Andrew Ward
In-house editors: Roisin O'Brien and Emma Hawkridge
Cover design: Tom Gordon

© 2003 Remedica Publishing Limited
All rights reserved. No part of this publication may be reproduced, stored in a retrieval system or transmitted in
any form or by any means, electronic, mechanical, photocopying, recording or otherwise, without the prior permission
of the publisher.

ISBN 1 901346 04 8
British Library Cataloguing-in Publication Data
A catalogue record for this book is available from the British Library

WITHDRAWN

SEXUAL HEALTH

in Obstetrics and Gynecology

Janet Wilson
Marian Everett

Editor:
James Walker

Lanchester Library

WITHDRAWN

REMEDICA
publishing

LONDON • CHICAGO

Contributors

Dr Janet Wilson, MB ChB, FRCP
Leeds General Infirmary
Leeds
UK

Dr Marian Everett, MB ChB, MFFP
Burmantofts Health Centre
Leeds
UK

Professor James Walker, MD, FRCP, FRCOG
St. James University Hospital
Leeds
UK

Coventry University

Contents

Foreword

In Britain today, sex is freely discussed almost everywhere, and particularly in the media. The pressure on young people to experiment with sex is greater than ever. The average age at first intercourse is steadily falling and in some surveys it is now lower than the legal age of consent.

Many countries have experienced similar changes, but Britain's sexual health – its teenage conception rate in particular – compares badly with other Western European nations. In recent years, the UK rates of chlamydial infection and viral sexually transmitted diseases have risen sharply, as has the abortion rate even though it is more than 40 years since the introduction of the oral contraceptive pill.

Sex education, having been neglected for a long time, is only just beginning to catch up with these social trends. Encouragingly, national initiatives to improve sexual health are now being supported at the highest level but there is still a long way to go. One teenager, quoted in a government report, said: "*It sometimes seems as if sex is compulsory but contraception is illegal.*"

Meanwhile, doctors in clinics up and down the country are faced with the challenge of trying to deliver high-quality care with small numbers of staff. Their work includes aspects of both gynecology and genitourinary medicine. Each of these specialties is traditionally self-contained but, as far as patients and diseases are concerned, there is no boundary between them.

The authors of this book are experienced doctors who know, first hand, the problems faced by practitioners in this field. They both work in an inner city. One is a consultant in a genitourinary medicine clinic and the other is a senior clinical medical officer in family planning, working in the hospital and in the community. Each devotes time and energy to teaching and research in addition to her busy clinical workload.

They have recognized the need for a book that covers all aspects of sexual health, and their collaboration has resulted in a text that is both practical and soundly based on evidence. The best medical textbooks are written by good teachers with a wealth of practical experience. This one is no exception.

James Owen Drife, MD, FRCOG, FRCPEd, FRCSEd, HonFCOGSA
Professor of Obstetrics and Gynaecology
University of Leeds, UK

chapter 1

Epidemiology of sexual health

Janet Wilson & Marian Everett

Epidemiology of sexually transmitted infections

Sexually transmitted infections (STIs) are one of the most common causes of illness in the world. Those in their reproductive years, who are economically the most productive, are predominantly affected. The long-term complications of STIs have a disproportionate effect on women, who are the bearers and usually the carers of children. STIs have a major impact on health, society, and the economy. In 1995, the World Health Organization (WHO) estimated that there were over 333 million cases of the four major curable STIs worldwide (with 90% occurring in developing countries) in the 15–49 age group [1]. In order of frequency these were:

- trichomoniasis (167.2 million cases)
- chlamydia (89.1 million cases)
- gonorrhea (62.2 million cases)
- syphilis (12.2 million cases)

In 2000, the WHO and the Joint United Nations Program on human immunodeficiency virus (HIV)/acquired immunodeficiency syndrome (AIDS) (UNAIDS) estimated that 36 million adults and children were living with HIV/AIDS (20 million people have already died as a result of the condition). About 95% live in developing countries, with two thirds estimated to be in Africa and a quarter in Asia. Cases of asymptomatic HIV infection have risen by 24% over the past 10 years in the UK. The number of males infected has been consistently higher than females, but the male to female ratio of new diagnoses has been steadily declining from 7.6:1 in 1990 to 1.9:1 in 1999 [2].

A substantial number of HIV infections in STI clinic attendees remain undiagnosed. In 1999, only 58% of heterosexual women in London who were found to be HIV-positive by unlinked anonymous prevalence monitoring had been diagnosed clinically. The Department of Health's National Health Strategy for Sexual Health and HIV has set a target of a 50% reduction in undiagnosed HIV-positive people by 2007. This is to be achieved by increasing HIV testing in STI clinics [3].

The prevalence of HIV infection in pregnant women has been increasing. One in 120 of those undergoing termination of pregnancy and 1 in 400 of antenatal clinic attendees were HIV-positive in 1999. This is a 6-fold increase since 1988 [4].

With the introduction of widespread HIV testing of pregnant women, the rate of maternal HIV diagnosis has improved. In 1999, 76% of pregnant women in inner London had their HIV infection diagnosed before delivery, compared with 50% in 1998 [4]. In the UK, a large proportion of heterosexually transmitted HIV infections are associated with having lived in or visited countries in sub-Saharan Africa. It is likely that the rapidly increasing rates of HIV infection in eastern Europe, Russia, other countries of the former USSR, and the Indian subcontinent will soon be reflected in the UK.

In western Europe, North America, and Australasia there was a steady decline in most bacterial STIs during the 1980s, but cases of viral STIs and chlamydia increased. In the late 1980s, this reduction in the UK, and other countries with access to early detection and STI treatment services, was further reduced by AIDS control programs promoting changes in sexual behavior and risk reduction. Chlamydia control programs have also reduced chlamydia infections in Nordic countries and areas of the USA and Canada.

Since the mid 1990s, the downward trend in bacterial STIs has started to reverse. In the UK, between 1995–1999, cases of chlamydia have risen by 76% (see Figure 1.1), gonorrhea by 55% (see Figure 1.2), and infectious syphilis by 54% [2]. Rises have been highest among teenagers and are likely to be a result of increasing unsafe sexual behavior. These rises, coupled with the continuing increase in the incidence of viral STIs (see Figures 1.3 and 1.4), put further strain on the already limited public STI healthcare services. The delay in treatment that may result prolongs the time over which the individual is infected, which in turn increases the transmission rate. Further public health campaigns are now needed in an attempt to reverse this pattern again. Cost-effective modeling has repeatedly indicated that targeted interventions, focusing on core risk groups rather than the general population, are the most cost-effective method and have the greatest impact on STI control. Plans for a national information campaign and targeted prevention campaigns are outlined in the National Strategy for Sexual Health and HIV [3].

Demographic factors associated with an increased risk of contracting and transmitting an STI are:

- age (peak incidence: 15–24 age group)
- being single, separated, or divorced
- using non-barrier contraception
- having an occupation that involves staying away from home

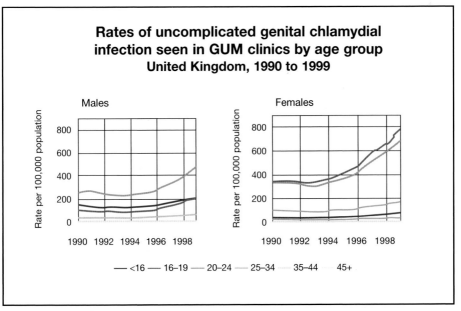

Figure 1.1 Increasing cases of chlamydia. With permission from the Public Health Laboratory Services [2].

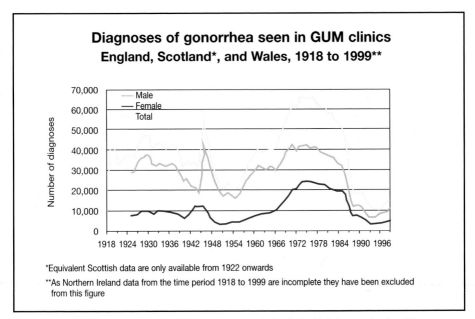

Figure 1.2 Increasing cases of gonorrhea. With permission from the Public Health Laboratory Services [2].

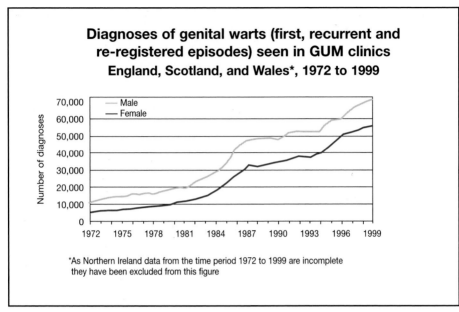

Figure 1.3 Increasing cases of genital warts. With permission from the Public Health Laboratory Services [2].

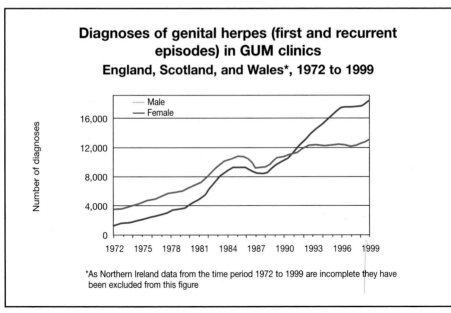

Figure 1.4 Increasing cases of genital herpes. With permission from the Public Health Laboratory Services [2].

In reality, these are surrogate markers of sexual activity and partner change rates. Knowledge of an individual's sexual history is essential to accurately assess his or her risk of having an STI.

The relationship between STIs and the use of contraception

Contraception can prevent unplanned pregnancy, with some forms also protecting against STIs. Unfortunately, the contraceptives with the lowest pregnancy rates provide minimal STI protection. Some contraceptives actually increase the risk of catching, and in turn transmitting, an infection. Before the advent of HIV/AIDS, most contraceptive policies tended to downplay the risks of STIs compared to those of unplanned pregnancy. HIV prevention programs placed great emphasis on condom use, possibly to the detriment of unplanned pregnancies. A solution to this problem is to encourage dual methods, one for pregnancy prevention and the other for STI/HIV protection. However, studies suggest that the more effective the primary method of contraception is, the lower the rate of consistent condom use becomes.

Male condoms, used correctly and consistently, protect both sexes against STIs and HIV. Female condoms may also protect, if they stay in position during intercourse. Barrier methods, such as the diaphragm used with spermicide, may also offer some protection, particularly against organisms such as chlamydia and gonorrhea that are transmitted between the male urethra and the cervix.

Combined oral contraception (COC) is associated with an increased risk of cervical infection with gonorrhea and chlamydia. This is probably because of the increased size of the cervical ectopy [5]. However, COC does protect against severe pelvic inflammatory disease (PID) requiring hospitalization, because it reduces the symptoms of upper genital tract infection [6]. Whether this represents a true protection against PID is unclear because, although COC reduces upper genital tract infection symptoms, it appears to increase the risk of unrecognized endometritis [7]. If COC users do develop PID, the inflammatory reaction of the Fallopian tubes tends to be less intense than in non-users [8]. Consequently, the fertility prognosis after PID is more favorable in COC users [9]. There are conflicting reports, but it appears that there might be a small but significant increased risk of acquiring HIV infection while using COC [10,11]. Studies looking at the link between injectable hormones and acquiring HIV infection have likewise suggested a small increased risk [11].

The intrauterine device (IUD) has an associated increased risk of PID within the first month after insertion [12], and a several-fold increased risk of bacterial vaginosis [13]. Early research indicated that prior IUD usage resulted in a 2- to 3-fold increased risk of tubal infertility and ectopic pregnancy, suggesting increased rates of PID in IUD users [14,15]. However, recent reviews have shown that the PID rate is similar, with or without an IUD, in women with asymptomatic gonorrhea or chlamydia. Furthermore, using an IUD does not affect tubal fertility [15]. When compared with non-hormonal IUDs, the progesterone implanted intrauterine system protects against salpingitis [17]. Sterilization offers no protection against catching an STI or HIV, but it does reduce the risk of PID [18].

Epidemiology of births, pregnancies, and deaths

At the end of 1999, the world population was estimated to be approximately 6 billion. The United Nations has predicted that the global population could be as high as 11 billion by the year 2050 [19]. There are about 185 million pregnancies per year and, of these, 45 million are terminated [20]. Approximately 78 000 women die each year from unsafe abortion worldwide [21].

In England and Wales around 190 000 abortions are carried out each year. The majority of these are in women between the ages of 20–29 (see Table 1.1).

Age category	<15	15	16–19	20–24	25–29	30–34	35–39	40–44	>45
no. of cases	1020	2414	29 947	44 960	40 159	28 892	16 858	5413	482

Table 1.1 Office for National Statistics 1997 abortion figures for women in England and Wales [22].

In England there are approximately 90 000 teenage conceptions per year. In 1997, the conception rate in under 16 year olds was 8.9 per 1000 (see Figure 1.5) [23]. These figures are the highest in Europe, with approximately 7500 conceptions annually in this age group resulting in 3700 live births. In total there are 56 000 live births and 34 000 terminations carried out in the UK teenage population each year [24]. In 1996 the UK birth rate in the 15–19 age group was the highest rate in Western Europe (see Figure 1.6) [25]. The target of the National Strategy on Teenage Pregnancy is to halve the teenage pregnancy rate by the year 2010.

By the age of 20, most individuals in the western World have had sexual intercourse. A study by Welling in 1995 [26] looked at the sexual attitudes and lifestyles of nearly 19 000 British residents aged between 16–59 years. Findings showed that the age of

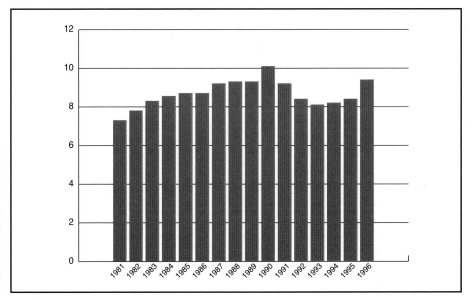

Figure 1.5 Conceptions in girls aged under 16 rose in 1996 for the third year running in England and Wales. With permission from BMJ [23].

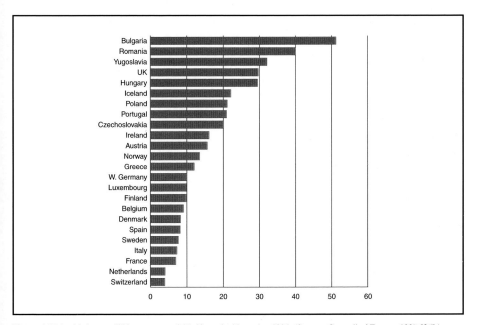

Figure 1.6 Live births per 1000 women aged 15–19, ranked by order, 1996. (Source: Council of Europe 1997 [25].)

first intercourse had fallen by 4 years for women and 3 years for men, to 17 in both sexes, over 4 decades. Of the cohort aged between 55–59 years, only 1% of females and 6% of males remembered having first sexual intercourse under the age of 16. The age of first sexual intercourse appears to be getting lower. A recent study of 1500 secondary school children by Burack [27] stated that 20% of 13 year olds reported having sexual intercourse or oral sex.

Use of contraception by teenagers

In 1999, a study on teenage pregnancy reported that 50% of sexually active under 16 year olds claimed that they had not used contraception the first time they had intercourse [28]. Burack reported that 19% of teenagers felt that they could not get pregnant as a result of first sexual intercourse, and 15% stated that they would have sex without using any contraception given the opportunity [27].

Teenagers who become sexually active before the age of 16 are more likely to take risks [29]. They tend to have more sexual partners in their lifetime and start sexual activity earlier in relationships than teenagers who become sexually active after the age of 16 [26,30]. Given the extent of the problems associated with teenage sexual activity – teenage conceptions, abortions, and the spread of STIs – a change in attitude and culture is necessary if any intervention is going to be successful.

References

1. Gerbase AC, Rowley JT, Heymann DH et al. Global prevalence and incidence estimates of selected curable STDs. *Sex Transm Infect* 1998;74(Suppl. 1):S12–6.

2. PHLS, DHSS&PS and the Scottish ISD(D)5 Collaborative Group. Trends in sexually transmitted infections in the United Kingdom 1990–1999. London: Public Health Laboratory Service, 2000.

3. The National Strategy for Sexual Health and HIV. Implementation action plan. London: Department of Health, 2002. Available at: URL: http://www.doh.gov.uk/sexualhealthandhiv/pdfs/77007betterpresersex.pdf

4. Unlinked Anonymous Surveys Steering Group (UASSG). Prevalence of HIV and Hepatitis Infections in the United Kingdom, 1999. London: Department of Health, Public Health Laboratory Service, Institute of Child Health, Scottish Centre for Infection and Environmental Health, 2000.

5. Louv WC, Austin H, Perlman J et al. Oral contraceptive use and risk of chlamydia and gonococcal infections. *Am J Obstet Gynecol* 1989;160:396–402.

6. Panser LA, Phipps WR. Type of oral contraceptive in relation to acute, initial episodes of pelvic inflammatory disease. *Contraception* 1991;43:91–9.

7. Ness RB, Keder LM, Soper DE et al. Oral contraception and the recognition of endometritis. *Am J Obstet Gynecol* 1997;176:580–5.

8. Wolner-Hanssen P, Eschenbach DA, Paavonen J et al. Decreased risk of symptomatic chlamydial pelvic inflammatory disease associated with oral contraceptive use. *JAMA* 1990;263:54–9.

9.   Westrom L, Joesoef R, Reynolds G et al. Pelvic inflammatory disease and infertility. A cohort study of 1,844 women with laparoscopically verified disease and 657 control women with normal laparoscopic results. *Sex Transm Dis* 1992;19:185–92.

10. Plummer FA, Simonsen JN, Cameron DW et al. Cofactors in male-female sexual transmission of human immunodeficiency virus type 1. *J Infect Dis* 1991;163:233–9.

11. Martin HL Jr, Nyange PM, Richardson BA et al. Hormonal contraception, sexually transmitted diseases, and risk of heterosexual transmission of human immunodeficiency virus type 1. *J Infect Dis* 1998;178:1053–9.

12. Buchan H, Villard-Mackingtosh L, Vessey M et al. Epidemiology of pelvic inflammatory disease in parous women with special reference to intrauterine device use. *Br J Obstet Gynaecol* 1990;97:780–8.

13. Moi H. Prevalence of bacterial vaginosis and its association with genital infections, inflammation and contraceptive methods in women attending sexually transmitted disease and primary health clinics. *Int J STD AIDS* 1990;1:86–94.

14. Daling JR, Weiss NS, Voigt LF et al. The intrauterine device and primary tubal infertility. *N Engl J Med* 1992;326:203–4.

15. Rossing MA, Daling JR, Weiss NS et al. Past use of an intrauterine device and risk of tubal pregnancy. *Epidemiology* 1993;4:245–51.

16. Grimes DA. Intrauterine device and upper genital tract infection. *Lancet* 2000;356:1013–9.

17. Luukkainen T, Toivonen J. Levonorgestrel-releasing IUD as a method of contraception with therapeutic properties. *Contraception* 1995;52:269–76.

18. Vessey M, Huggins G, Lawless M et al. Tubal sterilization: Findings in a large prospective study. *Br J Obstet Gynaecol* 1983;90:203–9.

19. Marwick C. US healthcare system too geared to acute medicine. *BMJ* 2001;322:572.

20. Guillebaud J. Contraception: Your Questions Answered. 3rd ed. Edinburgh: Churchill Livingstone, 1999.

21. Division of Reproductive Health, WHO. Unsafe abortion. Global and Regional Estimates of Incidence of and Mortality due to Unsafe Abortion. 3rd Ed. 1997. Available at: URL: http://www.who.int/reproductive-health/publications/MSM_97_16/MSM_97_16_table_of_contents_en.html

22. The Office for National Statistics. Legal abortions carried out under the 1967 Abortion Act in England and Wales, 1997. Abortion statistics AB no. 24. London: The Stationery Office.

23. Wise J. Teenage pregnancies rise in England and Wales. *BMJ* 1998;316:882.

24. Dickinson R, Fullerton D, Eastwood A et al. Effective Healthcare Bulletin – preventing and reducing the effects of unintended teenage pregnancies. NHS Centre for Review and Dissemination, University of York, 1997.

25. Council of Europe. Recent demographic developments in Europe – 1997. 1st edition. Council of Europe Publishing, 1997.

26. Wellings K, Wadsworth J, Johnson AM et al. Sexual attitudes and lifestyles. Oxford: Blackwell Scientific, 1994.

27. Burack R. Teenage sexual behaviour: attitudes towards and declared sexual activity. *Br J Fam Plan* 1999;24:145–8.

28. The Social Exclusion Unit. Teenage pregnancy report, no.cmnd 4342. London: The Stationery Office, 1999.

29. Mellanby A, Phelps F, Tripp J. Teenagers, sex and risk taking. *BMJ* 1993;307:683.

30. Curtis HA, Lawrence CJ, Tripp JH. Teenage sexual intercourse and pregnancy. *Arch Dis Child* 1988;63:373–9.

chapter 2

Sexual history, genital examination, and specimen taking in females

Janet Wilson

Many infections of the female genital tract, particularly those that are more serious, are asymptomatic. Even when symptoms are present, they are usually non-specific. Genital symptoms offer very few clues as to the location of the initial site of infection. All women presenting with genital symptoms need to be considered as possibly having a sexually transmitted infection (STI), and the likelihood of this needs to be assessed by taking a sexual history. A woman complaining of genital symptoms usually expects to have a related history taken so will not be offended as long as she is questioned in an appropriate and sensitive manner. The important questions to ask when taking a sexual history are provided in Tables 2.1 and 2.2.

A woman complaining of genital symptoms expects to be examined, and will usually be cooperative during the examination. Efforts from the examiner such as explaining the procedure to the woman, being aware of patient dignity, and performing the

---

The most recent sexual exposure

- when was it?
- was it a regular or casual partner?
- how long has there been a relationship with that person?
- what kind of contraception/protection was used?
- if condoms were used, were they used consistently and properly and were there any recent breakages?
- does the sexual partner have any genital symptoms?

A previous sexual partner

- how long has it been since sex with a different partner?
- if within the past few months the same details as above need to be obtained

How many different partners have there been over the past few months?

Table 2.1 Questions to ask when taking a sexual history.

Has the patient ever injected drugs?

Have there been any high-risk male partners?

- bisexual men?
- injecting drug users?
- men from areas of high HIV prevalence, e.g. sub-Saharan Africa and Asia?

If yes to any of the above, when was the most recent exposure?

Table 2.2 Questions to assess the risk of HIV infection.

The female genital examination should include:

- inspection of the pubic hair and surrounding skin for pediculosis pubis, molluscum contagiosum, and dermatological conditions
- inguinal palpation for lymphadenopathy
- inspection of the labia majora, minora, clitoris, introitus (to do this the labia need to be separated), perineum, and perianal area for warts, ulcers, erythema, excoriation, or visible discharge
- inspection of the urethral meatus and the Skene's and Bartholin's glands
- insertion of a bivalve speculum; a lubricant should not be applied to the speculum as this can interfere with microbiological tests, instead the speculum can be warmed and lubricated with warm water
- inspection of the vaginal walls for erythema, discharge, warts, or ulcers
- inspection of the cervix for discharge, erythema, contact bleeding, ulcers, or raised lesions
- bimanual pelvic examination to assess size and any tenderness of the uterus, cervical motion tenderness, adnexal tenderness, or masses

Table 2.3 The female examination for detection of genital infections.

examination with minimal discomfort will maintain cooperation and enhance the chances of obtaining useful specimens. Simple considerations such as warming the speculum add greatly to the woman's comfort during the examination. The examiner should also take into account ethnic and sexuality issues (e.g. some women prefer not to be examined by a male doctor) and be aware of the need for a chaperone. The important aspects of the examination for genital infections are described in Table 2.3.

To make a correct diagnosis of the cause of female genital infections:

- perform a urethral culture for gonorrhea
- collect a first-pass urine sample for a chlamydia DNA amplification test. If an enzyme immunoassay (EIA) is the only detection technique available, take a urethral sample
- look at the vaginal discharge to see if it has a homogenous, white appearance
- perform a vaginal pH test using narrow-range pH paper. The vaginal swab can be touched onto the paper or the paper can be pressed against the lateral vaginal walls with sponge holders. It is important that cervical secretions are avoided as cervical mucus has a pH of 7 and any contamination will give a falsely high reading
- perform a vaginal amine 'whiff' test by mixing a loop of vaginal secretions with 10% potassium hydroxide on a glass slide. The mixture should be smelt immediately for the characteristic transient 'dead fish' odor
- if on-site microscopy is available, take a wet-mount slide by placing a loop of vaginal secretions in a drop of saline then examine by phase contrast microscopy. Alternatively, take a vaginal smear for Gram staining in the laboratory. Both the wet-mount and Gram-stained slides should be examined for clue cells (vaginal epithelial cells covered in the bacteria that make up bacterial vaginosis), pseudohyphae, and spores. About 50% of candida infections can be diagnosed this way
- perform a candida culture and a *Trichomonas vaginalis* culture (these are likely to be taken on the same vaginal sample and sent to the laboratory in transport medium)
- perform an endocervical culture for gonorrhea
- take an endocervical sample for a chlamydia DNA amplification test. Perform an EIA if this is the only detection technique available
- if vesicles, ulcers, or fissures are found, a sample for herpes culture should be taken from the base of the lesion and sent to the laboratory in viral transport medium
- take a blood sample for syphilis serology
- take a blood sample for HIV testing if the patient gives informed consent
- offer hepatitis B testing if the patient, or any of her sexual partners, is from an area with high hepatitis B prevalence (sub-Saharan Africa and Asia). If testing is negative, offer hepatitis B immunization
- offer hepatitis B and C testing (and hepatitis B immunization) if the patient, or any of her sexual partners, has previously injected drugs

Table 2.4 Summary of specimens taken to diagnose female genital infections.

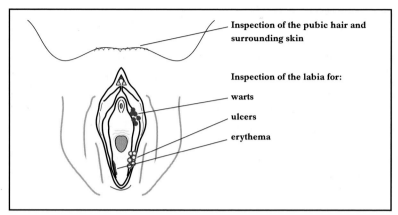

Inspection of the pubic hair and surrounding skin

Inspection of the labia for:

warts

ulcers

erythema

Figure 2.1 External examination of the female genitalia.

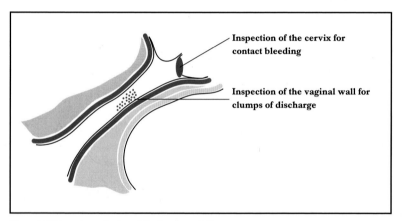

Inspection of the cervix for contact bleeding

Inspection of the vaginal wall for clumps of discharge

Figure 2.2 Internal examination of the female genitalia.

It is important that the examination is thorough. Unfortunately, failure to detect the different clinical signs of specific genital infections in women may be due to poor clinical skills or reluctance by the examiner to perform an adequate genital examination. Women with symptoms suggestive of a genital tract infection should be examined. Figures 2.1 and 2.2 demonstrate how the external and internal female genitalia examinations should be performed and how specimens should be taken.

Specimens should be collected during the examination (see Table 2.4). When taking swabs it is important that the procedure is carried out correctly and that the specimen is placed in the appropriate culture or transport medium. Further details are given in the relevant sections about specific infections in the following chapters.

When taking urethral and endocervical samples, it is important to obtain cellular material. For an endocervical specimen, a swab needs to be placed 1 cm into the endocervical canal. It should then be rotated vigorously for about 10 seconds before being placed in medium. For a urethral specimen, a fine swab should be inserted gently into the urethral opening. It should be rotated gently through about 180 degrees before being placed into medium. To reduce the cost of microbiological tests, the urethral and endocervical samples for gonorrhea testing can be placed in the same container and can be processed together. This is also true for chlamydia testing of urethral and endocervical samples.

As the blood tests for HIV and hepatitis C are based on the detection of antibodies, it can take up to 3 months for the tests to become positive after infection. This is sometimes referred to as the 'window period'. There can be a similar delay in the detection of hepatitis B. If the patient has had possible exposure to these infections within the past 3 months, she should be advised to have a further blood test in 3 months' time. The management of HIV and hepatitis B and C infections is not covered in this book. Referral should be made to a specialist unit.

chapter 3

Vulval and urethral problems

Janet Wilson

Vulval problems

There are a number of conditions that can present with vulval symptoms and signs. These can be broadly divided into conditions causing vulval lumps, ulcers, and irritation (see Table 3.1).

Vulval lumps	Vulval ulcers	Vulval irritation
Genital warts	Genital herpes	Candida infections
Molluscum contagiosum	Primary syphilis	*Trichomonas vaginalis*
Syphilitic condylomata lata	Behçet's syndrome	Pediculosis pubis
Normal sebaceous glands		Irritant vulvitis
Vulval papillae		Lichen simplex
Sebaceous cysts		Vulval eczema
Vulval intra-epithelial neoplasia		Vulval psoriasis
		Vulval lichen sclerosus
Vulval cancer		Vulval lichen planus
Skene's (periurethral) gland abscess		Atrophic vulvitis
Bartholin's gland abscess		

Table 3.1 The main causes of vulval problems.

VULVAL LUMPS

Genital warts are by far the most common cause of vulval lumps. Like genital warts, molluscum contagiosum and condylomata lata are caused by infections and are usually painless. Skene's (periurethral) and Bartholin's gland abscesses may present as painful vulval lumps. These may be caused by gonorrhea or chlamydial infections. Prominent vulval sebaceous glands and papillae are normal anatomical variants.

Genital warts

Prevalence rates

Genital warts are the most common sexually transmitted infection (STI) in Europe and the US. Epidemiological studies suggest that human papillomavirus (HPV) can be detected in the genital region of 20%–25% of women between the ages of 18–25 years, but only about 1% of these women will develop clinically evident warts. A cohort study of human immunodeficiency virus-negative (HIV-negative) women in the US reported a baseline prevalence of genital warts of 1.2%. During follow-up, the incidence was shown to be 0.8 per 100 person years [1]. In 1999, 61 559 new patients presented with genital warts to genitourinary medicine (GUM) clinics in England. First attack, recurrent, and re-registered cases of genital warts accounted for 21% of all diagnoses made [2].

Etiology

Genital warts are painless, benign, epithelial tumors. Most cases of genital warts are caused by HPV type 6 (HPV-6), with some being caused by HPV type 11 (HPV-11) infection. These viral subtypes can cause:

- latent infection
- subclinical infection
- clinically apparent benign warts
- low-grade cervical intra-epithelial neoplasia

The HPV types that cause genital warts are mucus membrane specific, so they are almost always sexually transmitted. Occasionally, common wart types can be autoinoculated onto the thighs, pubic region, and labia majora, but these warts are unable to grow on mucus membranes. Genital warts are often associated with other more serious STIs such as chlamydia. One study found that 18% of women with genital warts also had chlamydia and 25% had at least one other STI [3].

Genital warts are highly infectious. Two thirds of partners will themselves develop warts. Using DNA detection techniques, up to 94% of partners have been found to have latent HPV infection. The average incubation period is 3 months but it can extend to years.

Clinical manifestations

Genital warts are painless. In women they may not be noticed by the patient: they are often detected during a genital examination for something else. They can be single, but are usually multiple. They typically appear at areas of minor abrasion during sex, i.e.

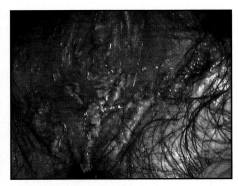

Figure 3.1 Clinical picture of genital warts.

around the introital opening and hymen remnants (see Figure 3.1). They then spread onto the labia, perineum, and perianal area. On the mucus membranes they are usually soft and cauliflower-like (condylomata acuminata), whereas on the drier surfaces they are harder, keratinized, and papular. These papular lesions can be pigmented.

Diagnosis
Genital warts are diagnosed by their clinical appearance. Any lesion that is atypical should be biopsied, particularly in older women, as premalignant and malignant lesions can look similar.

Management
Guidelines for the management of anogenital warts are provided by Maw [4]. Warts can sometimes regress spontaneously but are more likely to enlarge, proliferate, and persist without treatment. No single treatment is ideal for all patients or all warts.

Topical podophyllotoxin can be used to treat multiple, soft warts (condylomata acuminata). This derivative of podophyllin is available for home treatment as a 0.5% solution or a 0.15% cream. It is applied twice daily for 3 consecutive days per week for up to 4 weeks. It acts as a cytotoxic agent, so is contraindicated during pregnancy as it may have a teratogenic effect.

For fewer or keratinized warts, an ablative treatment such as cryotherapy, trichloroacetic acid, curettage, or electrocautery is usually chosen. Cryotherapy, using liquid nitrogen or nitrous oxide, can be safely used on all warts including those in the urethra. It should be used weekly and is safe to use during pregnancy. Trichloroacetic acid (80%–90% solution) is highly corrosive. It should be applied carefully to the warts (as it can cause local skin ulceration) by medical or nursing staff on a weekly basis. It can be used safely during pregnancy. Removal under local anesthetic by curettage or diathermy excision is very effective for small numbers of pedunculated warts and it has the added benefits of potentially treating the patient in a single session and having a relatively low recurrence rate. Electrosurgery or laser therapy under general anesthetic is sometimes used for recalcitrant warts.

All treatments may have recurrence rates of up to 25%. The reason for this high recurrence is that treatments remove the warts but do not clear the surrounding subclinical viral infection.

Imiquimod cream is a relatively new wart treatment. It is an immune modulator that boosts local cellular immunity resulting in wart clearance. It can be used on both soft and keratinized warts. It is a home treatment that is applied daily on alternate days for up to 16 weeks. It has lower recurrence rates compared to most other treatments but it may take several weeks before a clinical response is recognized. It should not be used during pregnancy.

All women with genital warts should be tested for other STIs. It is usually advised that sexual partners are also examined for genital warts and tested for other STIs. The initiation of condom use in a longstanding sexual relationship is likely to offer little protection as the partner will probably already have been infected. However, patients should be advised to use condoms with any new sexual partner. Genital warts are not an indication for increased cervical cytology screening [5].

Recurrent infections
After apparently clearing, warts will recur in about 25% of cases. This is because the subclinical infection persists and can later produce clinical lesions. A person's immune response most probably determines whether an HPV infection becomes clinically manifest, how favorably the warts respond to any treatment, and whether they recur. As imiquimod stimulates local cell-mediated immunity, it may be more effective than other treatments for recurrent warts.

Complications
Complications from HPV-6 and HPV-11 are rare. Very occasionally they can induce the formation of Buschke–Loewenstein giant condyloma, a locally invasive but non-metastasizing tumor. Although rare, vertical transmission can occur. Women with genital warts frequently have subclinical cervical HPV-6 and HPV-11 infections, which may present as low-grade cervical abnormalities. However, studies investigating the incidence of cervical cancer or high-grade abnormalities have reported no significant

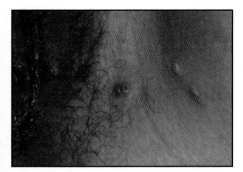

Figure 3.2 Clinical picture of molluscum contagiosum.

increase in women with a history of genital warts [6]. Consequently, in the UK, the Cervical Screening Program recommends normal interval screening for women with genital warts [5]. The main morbidity associated with genital warts is psychological. A number of studies have reported high levels of depression and diminished sexual function [7].

Molluscum contagiosum

Etiology
This benign papular infection, caused by the molluscum contagiosum virus, can be sexually transmitted in adults if present on the genital area. The virus is transmitted by direct skin-to-skin contact. The incubation period is 2–3 months. An overview of this condition is provided by Scott [8].

Clinical manifestations
Initially, papules are skin colored and usually multiple. They enlarge to a diameter of 3–5 mm, but may occasionally reach 10–15 mm. They then become umbilicated, i.e. they develop a central pit (see Figure 3.2) from which caseous material can be squeezed. They are usually present on the lower abdomen, thigh, and genital area. They are painless unless they become secondarily infected. No complications have been described.

Diagnosis
The diagnosis is made on the clinical appearance.

Management
Generally, the lesions cause few problems and often clear spontaneously. People with genital molluscum contagiosum often have other STIs so testing for other infections should be performed. If therapy is required lesions can be treated using mechanical

destruction techniques such as trichloroacetic acid, cryotherapy, or removal of the central core. Podophyllotoxin cream as a home treatment has also been shown to be effective [8].

VULVAL ULCERS

The main cause of vulval ulceration in Europe is genital herpes. Until recently, infective syphilis was extremely rare, but in recent years several outbreaks of early infectious syphilis have been reported in England. It is therefore important to remain vigilant and perform syphilis serology on all women with vulval ulceration.

Genital herpes
Prevalence rates
The rates of genital herpes are rising throughout the world. In the UK, there was a 6-fold increase in the number of cases between 1972–1994. Herpes simplex virus type 2 (HSV-2) antibodies have been detected in 7.6% of blood donors and in approximately 20% of STI clinic attendees. Less than half of those with detectable HSV-2 antibodies have a clinical history of herpes, suggesting that many people acquire subclinical infection. HSV-1 cases are increasing, particularly in young women. This is probably due to increasing orogenital sex.

Etiology
Genital herpes can be caused by either HSV-1 or HSV-2. HSV-1 is usually the cause of orolabial herpes (cold sores) and between 30%–50% of genital herpes. HSV-2 is responsible for the remaining cases of genital herpes but rarely causes cold sores.

The natural history of genital herpes is complex. Following inoculation of the mucosa, the HSV ascends the peripheral sensory nerves and enters the dorsal root ganglion where latency is established. From time to time it can reactivate producing recurrent lesions. During reactivation, lesions are not always noticeable; completely asymptomatic, subclinical viral shedding is well described. Even though these reactivated episodes may not be clinically evident, they are potentially infectious.

Clinical manifestations
Primary genital herpes
The primary infection is the first-ever exposure to either HSV-1 or HSV-2. It can be asymptomatic or may cause vulval soreness and external dysuria. Because of these non-specific symptoms it is often initially misdiagnosed as either a urinary tract or candida infection. There may also be systemic symptoms, characteristic of a flu-like illness. Vesicles may be detected on examination (see Figure 3.3) but these usually have already ruptured to form multiple painful ulcers on the vulva. The ulcers are

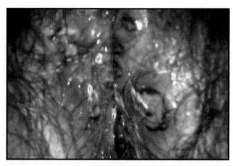

Figure 3.4 Clinical picture of herpes ulcers.

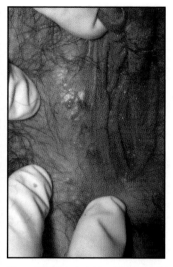

Figure 3.3 Clinical picture of herpes vesicles.

shallow with a thin rim of surrounding erythema (see Figure 3.4). Tender inguinal lymphadenopathy is usually evident. Without treatment, lesions increase in size and number over 7 days. After this period, crusting appears and the lesions gradually settle after 14–21 days. Latent infection, with the possibility of recurrence, occurs after both symptomatic and subclinical infections. Following the primary infection, viral antibodies can be detected.

Non-primary, first episode genital herpes
Non-primary, first-episode genital herpes occurs in people with previous orolabial HSV-1 who then acquire genital HSV-2 infection. There is some cross-protection from the previous HSV infection, which results in a milder illness. Such HSV-2 infections are asymptomatic more often than primary infections.

Recurrent herpes
Recurrent herpes occurs when the virus in the sensory ganglion is reactivated. The lesions occur in the area of skin innervated by that ganglion. Recurrences may be asymptomatic (subclinical shedding), but if symptoms are present they are usually milder and localized to a smaller area than with primary infection. They may be characterized by a prodrome of tingling, itching, or pain prior to the eruption of the vesicles. On examination there are usually just a few localized ulcers (see Figure 3.5). These heal within 6–12 days without treatment.

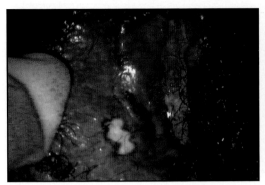

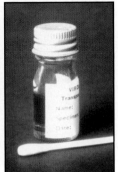

Figure 3.5 Clinical picture of recurrent herpes.　　　　**Figure 3.6** Herpes transport medium.

Within the first year of primary HSV-2 infection nearly all (90%) people will develop a recurrence. Some of these recurrences will be characterized by subclinical virus shedding. Both symptomatic and subclinical reactivations are less frequent (about 60% in the first year) with HSV-1 infections. The average recurrence rate is twice per year but in a few patients this may be more frequent. Long-term cohort studies indicate that the frequency of symptomatic recurrence gradually decreases with time.

Diagnosis
Even if the characteristic clinical appearance is suggestive of herpes, the diagnosis should be confirmed by viral culture. Although viral culture is still considered to be the 'gold standard', polymerase chain reaction is a more sensitive detection method for HSV (at present it is only used in research settings). The sample for culture should be taken from the base of the lesion as early in the outbreak as possible and sent to the laboratory in viral transport medium (see Figure 3.6). As HSV is a labile virus, the transport medium needs to be kept cool (4°C) and the sample needs to be transported rapidly to the laboratory. If these culture facilities are not available, the patient should be referred to a GUM or specialist STI service for accurate diagnosis.

HSV serology is only useful if it is type specific, i.e. if it can distinguish between HSV-1 and HSV-2 antibodies. Such tests are not yet widely available in the UK and there is debate over their place in patient management [9].

Management of the first clinical episode of genital herpes
Recommendations for the management of genital herpes are provided by the Herpes Simplex Advisory Panel [10]. Antiviral drugs used to treat a primary attack significantly reduce the severity and duration of symptoms, the time taken for the lesion to heal, and result in the cessation of viral shedding. These drugs are most

effective if treatment is initiated within 5 days of the appearance of symptoms. However, they do not prevent latency and therefore have no effect on future recurrences. Recommended treatment regimens are:

- aciclovir, 200 mg, five times daily for 5 days
- famciclovir, 250 mg, three times daily for 5 days
- valaciclovir, 500 mg, twice daily for 5 days

Aciclovir can be used during pregnancy and while breastfeeding.

Anti-inflammatory analgesia and saline bathing are both recommended as supportive measures. Patients can be advised to pass urine in a bath of warm water to ease external dysuria.

Other STIs may accompany primary genital herpes so testing for other infections is imperative. However, this can safely be deferred for a few days, allowing the vulval ulceration to heal before a vaginal speculum is inserted. Patients should be counseled regarding the natural history of the infection with emphasis on the potential for recurrent episodes, subclinical viral shedding, sexual transmission, and possible treatments.

Management of recurrent genital herpes
Recurrences are less severe than the primary episode; they are self-limiting and can often be managed by supportive therapy. Early episodic antiviral therapy will reduce the duration and severity of an attack but will not reduce the number of recurrences. This approach is therefore appropriate when recurrences are infrequent but severe. It is appropriate for the patient to initiate this treatment at home as soon as a recurrence is noticed. Episodic treatment regimens are:

- aciclovir, 200 mg, five times a day for 5 days
- famciclovir, 125 mg, twice daily for 5 days
- valaciclovir, 500 mg, twice daily for 5 days

Daily suppressive therapy can be used to reduce frequent recurrences. This is often reserved for patients with more than six recurrences in a year. Suppressive treatment regimens are:

- aciclovir, 400 mg, twice daily
- famciclovir, 250 mg, twice daily
- valaciclovir, 250 mg, twice daily
- valaciclovir 500 mg, once daily

The aciclovir regimen is the cheapest treatment available and has the longest safety record. It is usual to prescribe this treatment for 6–12 months. About 20% of patients will experience a reduction in the recurrence rate after stopping treatment. Treatment may be safely restarted if frequent recurrences persist.

Patients should be advised to avoid sexual contact during the prodrome and any recurrence, as this is when the risk of transmission is highest. They should also be advised that they are potentially infectious even when they have no obvious recurrence because of subclinical viral shedding. Condoms may reduce the risk of transmission but this has not been formally studied.

Complications
Herpes in pregnancy can be transmitted to the neonate. Women with primary genital herpes during pregnancy, particularly in the third trimester, are most at risk of vertical transmission. The risk of perinatal transmission with recurrent HSV appears to be low. The management of herpes in pregnancy is discussed in detail in Chapter 6.

Cohort studies have shown that prior HSV-2 infection increases the chance of contracting HIV by 2- to 3-fold [11]. Epidemiological data also suggest an increased transmission of HIV with herpes.

As genital herpes is a chronic, recurring condition, many people develop psychological sequelae. Studies have reported high levels of depression and fear of rejection by future partners.

Occasionally, with a primary infection, aseptic meningitis and autonomic neuropathy (leading to urinary retention) can occur. Occasionally, the infection can disseminate, causing a life-threatening condition. This is more likely in an immunocompromised patient and during pregnancy.

Syphilis
Prevalence rates
Until the 1990s, cases of infectious syphilis had dropped to such low levels in the UK that the need for antenatal screening for this infection was being questioned. However, throughout the mid to late 1990s there were several outbreaks with some cases only being detected as a result of antenatal screening. Consequently, syphilis screening in pregnancy remains cost-effective and should be continued [12].

Etiology
Syphilis is caused by the spirochete, *Treponema pallidum*. Humans are the only host and in adults the infection is sexually transmitted.

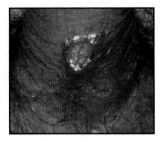

Figure 3.7 Clinical picture of the syphilitic chancre.

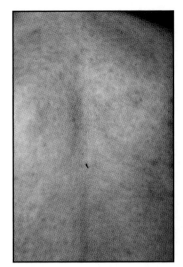

Figure 3.8 Clinical picture of the secondary syphilis rash.

Clinical manifestations

There are several stages of syphilis infection:

Primary syphilis

Approximately 10–90 (on average 21) days after exposure, a chancre appears at the site of infection. The chancre is usually a single, painless ulcer, about 1 cm in diameter with rolled indurated edges (see Figure 3.7). As the chancre is painless it usually goes unnoticed in women as it is often not visible. Regional lymphadenopathy is usually evident. If left untreated it heals spontaneously within a few weeks. Syphilis serology may still be negative at this stage of infection.

Secondary syphilis

After a few weeks or months, a generalized illness may develop, which is characterized by a low-grade fever and malaise with skin and mucosal rashes. The rash is typically maculopapular over the trunk, extremities, palms, and soles (see Figure 3.8). The lesions are reddish brown and are easily mistaken for psoriasis or pityriasis rosea. Wart-like moist papules occur on the mucosal surfaces of the genital tract (condylomata lata) and can sometimes also be seen in the axillae and in the groin (see Figure 3.9). Mucosal ulcerating lesions may be visible in the mouth. Without treatment these symptoms and signs will resolve after 3–12 weeks. Syphilis serology is strongly positive at this stage of the infection.

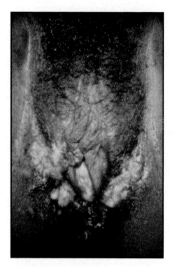

Figure 3.9 Clinical picture of condylomata lata of syphilis.

Late syphilis

Without treatment, up to 40% of patients will develop symptomatic late syphilis with neurosyphilis, cardiovascular syphilis, or gummata.

Diagnosis

The national guidelines for diagnosis and management are provided by Goh [13]. The spirochetes can be seen on samples from the chancre, lymph nodes, or genital mucosal lesions under dark-field microscopy. The easiest and most reliable way to diagnose syphilis is by serological testing. Some laboratories use enzyme immunoassay as the screening test. If positive, a Venereal Disease Research Laboratory test, rapid plasma reagin test, *Treponema pallidum* hemagglutination test, and fluorescent treponemal antibody absorption test should be performed.

Management

The treatment of syphilis requires long courses of antibiotics and long-term follow-up. Therefore, it should only be undertaken by specialists. The patient should be referred to a GUM or specialist STI service.

Complications

Without treatment, complications of late syphilis can occur. Syphilis in pregnancy can be transmitted to the infant (see Chapter 6).

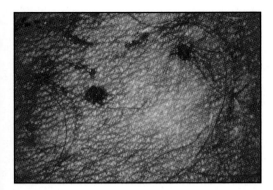

Figure 3.10 Clinical picture of pediculosis pubis.

VULVAL IRRITATION/ITCHING

There are a number of infective causes of vulval irritation. Candida infections and *Trichomonas vaginalis* infect the vagina but both can cause vulval irritation (see Chapter 4). Many women mistake their vulval symptoms for recurrent candida infections when in fact they have vulval dermatoses.

Pediculosis pubis (pubic lice)

Etiology

The crab louse, *Phthirus pubis*, is transmitted by body contact. The usual incubation period is between 5 days and a few weeks. An overview of this infection is provided by Scott [14].

Clinical manifestations

The main symptoms are irritation within the pubic hair area or the recognition of lice. The condition may also remain asymptomatic. There are no long-term complications from this infection.

Diagnosis

Clinical examination reveals the characteristic lice and eggs (see Figure 3.10). The nits are cemented onto the hair shaft, 1–2 mm above the skin. The lice may look like freckles or small scabs.

Management

A 1% permethrin cream rinse should be applied to damp hair and rinsed off after 10 minutes. It is safe to use during pregnancy and while breastfeeding. Testing for other STIs should be carried out and sexual partners should be examined and treated.

Vulval dermatoses

Etiology

There are a number of dermatological conditions that can present with vulval problems. These include irritant and allergic vulvitis, eczema, psoriasis, lichen simplex, lichen sclerosus, and lichen planus. There are several common aspects with regards to presentation and management.

Clinical manifestations

Common symptoms are vulval itching and soreness. On examination there may be erythema, lichenification, and fissuring in addition to the specific appearances associated with the condition.

Diagnosis

The diagnosis is made on the clinical appearance of the vulva and a general examination of the skin. A biopsy may be needed.

Management

Exclude candida infections. General advice for all vulval conditions is to avoid contact with soap and shampoo by using aqueous cream (BP) as a soap substitute and general emollient.

Urethral problems

DYSURIA

About 20% of women complain of dysuria each year. This symptom can usually be attributed to acute bacterial cystitis, urethritis, or vulvitis. There are a number of features relating to the history and examination that can help to distinguish between these sites of infection (see Table 3.2).

The incidence of acute bacterial cystitis is highest in sexually active women in the 20–25 age category. Sexual intercourse, the use of spermicides and diaphragms, a history of prior cystitis, and a recent course of antibiotics have been identified as independent risk factors. The diagnosis is made on mid-stream urine microscopy and culture. A study in young women suggested that the traditional diagnostic criterion of $\geq 10^5$ uropathogens per mL of urine was not sensitive enough for the diagnosis of acute bacterial cystitis, which presents with dysuria and frequency; the bacterial concentration can range from as little as 10^2 to 10^5 per mL [15]. This criterion was established in women with acute pyelonephritis. Almost all episodes of bacterial cystitis are accompanied by pyuria and there may be frank hematuria in up to 20% of cases. The common causal organisms are coliforms (80% of cases) and *Staphylococcus saprophyticus* (5%–15% of cases).

	Acute bacterial cystitis	**Urethritis**	**Vulvitis**
Causes	Coliform bacteria *Staphylococcus saprophyticus*	*Chlamydia trachomatis* *Neisseria gonorrhoeae*	Genital herpes Candida infections *Trichomonas vaginalis* All causes of vulval dermatoses
Symptoms	Internal dysuria Frequency and urgency Hematuria	Internal dysuria No hematuria Vaginal discharge	External dysuria Vaginal discharge Vulval irritation, burning, or pain
Signs	Suprapubic tenderness	Cervicitis	Vulval ulcers Vulvitis Vaginal discharge

Table 3.2 The causes, symptoms, and signs associated with dysuria.

The usual treatments for uncomplicated acute bacterial cystitis are [16]:

- a 3 day course of one of the following:

    trimethoprim, 200 mg, twice daily

    cephalexin, 500 mg, twice daily

    ciprofloxacin, 100 mg, twice daily

- a 7 day course of: nitrofurantoin, 50 mg, four times daily

Trimethoprim is usually a first-line treatment and is effective against about 70% of urinary pathogens. Approximately 15% of cases are resistant to nitrofurantoin, less than 10% are resistant to cephalosporins, and approximately 5% are resistant to ciprofloxacin [16].

Women are often referred to as having urethral syndrome when they present with dysuria, with or without frequency, but in the absence of a detectable urine infection. Many have sterile pyuria. Studies have shown that this is commonly caused by chlamydial infection. Gonorrhea can also cause urethritis so can similarly present as sterile pyuria. The diagnosis and management of these infections are covered in Chapter 4.

Although herpes infections are not a common cause of dysuria, the most common presenting symptom of primary herpes in women is external dysuria. If an examination is not performed, the vulval lesions will be missed. A herpes infection can commonly be mistaken for acute bacterial cystitis.

References

1.   Chirgwin K, Feldman J, Augenbraun M et al. Incidence of venereal warts in HIV-infected and uninfected women. *J Infect Dis* 1995;172:235–8.

2.   PHLS, DHSS&PS and the Scottish ISD(D)5 Collaborative Group. Trends in sexually transmitted infections in the United Kingdom 1990–1999. New episodes seen at genitourinary medicine clinics. London: Public Health Laboratory Service, 2000.

3.   Carne CA, Dockerty G. Genital warts: need to screen for coinfection. *BMJ* 1990;300:459.

4.   Maw R. National guideline for the management of anogenital warts. *Sex Transm Infect* 1999;75(Suppl. 1):S71–5.

5.   Duncan I, editor. Guidelines for clinical practice and programme management. 2nd Edition. London NHS Cervical Screening Programme Publication No 8. December, 1997.

6.   Sigurgeirsson B, Lindelof B, Eklund G. Condylomata acuminata and risk of cancer: an epidemiological study. *BMJ* 1991;303:341–4.

7.   Clarke P, Ebel C, Cototti DN et al. The psychosocial impact of human papillomavirus infection: implications for health care providers. *Int J STD AIDS* 1996;75:312–6.

8.   Scott G. National guideline for the management of molluscum contagiosum. *Sex Transm Infect* 1999;75(Suppl 1):S80–1.

9.   Cowen FM. Testing for type-specific antibody to herpes simplex virus – implications for clinical practice. *J Antimicrob Chemother* 2000;45(Suppl T3):9–13.

10.   Herpes Simplex Advisory Panel. National guideline for the management of genital herpes. *Sex Transm Infect* 1999;75(Suppl 1):S24–8.

11.   Dickerson MC, Johnston J, Delea TE et al. The causal role for genital ulcer disease as a risk factor for transmission of human immunodeficiency virus: an application of the Bradford Hill criteria. *Sex Transm Dis* 1996;23:429–40.

12.   Hurtig AK, Nicoll A, Carne C et al. Syphilis in pregnant women and their children in the United Kingdom: results from national clinician reporting surveys 1994–7. *BMJ* 1998;317:1617–9.

13.   Goh B. National guideline for the management of early syphilis. *Sex Transm Infect* 1999;75(Suppl. 1):S29–33.

14.   Scott G. National guideline for the management of *Phthirus pubis* infestation. *Sex Transm Infect* 1999;75(Suppl. 1):S78–9.

15.   Stamm WE, Counts GW, Running KR et al. Diagnosis of coliform infection in acutely dysuric women. *N Eng J Med* 1982;307:463–8.

16.   Winstanley TG, Limb DI, Eggington R et al. A 10 year survey of the antimicrobial susceptibility of urinary tract isolates in the UK: the Microbe Base project. *J Antimicrob Chemother* 1997;40:591–4.

chapter 4

Vaginal discharge

Janet Wilson

Vaginal discharge is a non-specific symptom. The causes range from serious infections like *Neisseria gonorrhoeae* and *Chlamydia trachomatis*, non-infective causes such as retained tampons, through to physiological discharge (see Table 4.1). Clinical signs and symptoms do not help to distinguish between vaginal and cervical infections. Bacterial vaginosis, candida infections, and *Trichomonas vaginalis* are vaginal infections whereas *C. trachomatis* and *N. gonorrhoeae* are cervical infections.

Infective	Non-infective
Bacterial vaginosis	Cervical ectropion
Candida infections	Cervical polyp
Chlamydia trachomatis	Retained tampons
Neisseria gonorrhoeae	Retained products of conception
Trichomonas vaginalis	Neoplasms

Table 4.1 The main causes of vaginal discharge. The infective causes are arranged in the order of frequency of occurrence.

Bacterial vaginosis

PREVALENCE RATES

This is the most common cause of vaginal discharge in women of reproductive age. Prevalence rates vary depending on the population being studied. The rates in the UK are about 9% in general practice, 15% in pregnant women, 20%–25% in women undergoing termination of pregnancy (TOP), and 30% in women attending sexually transmitted infection (STI) clinics. In African countries, studies have reported rates of over 50% [1].

ETIOLOGY

Bacterial vaginosis (BV) is caused by an overgrowth of anaerobic bacteria, genital mycoplasmas, and *Gardnerella vaginalis* (all of which can normally be present in small numbers in the vagina), with reduced or absent lactobacilli. Although

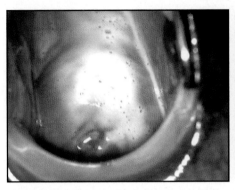

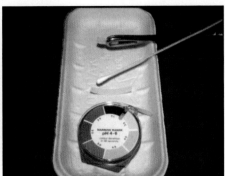

Figure 4.1 Clinical picture of bacterial vaginosis vaginal discharge.

Figure 4.2 Bacterial vaginosis and raised pH.

associated with an increased number of sexual partners, BV is not considered to be an STI. Randomized placebo-controlled studies have shown no decrease in recurrence when the male partner is treated.

Other known risk factors for BV are:

- smoking
- vaginal douching
- using an intrauterine device (IUD)

CLINICAL MANIFESTATIONS

It is thought that about 50% of women with BV are asymptomatic. When present, symptoms include increased vaginal discharge and malodor (the unpleasant smell is caused by the production of volatile amines by anaerobic bacteria). The odor is often worse after sexual intercourse (semen [pH 8] causes a further release of volatile amines) and during menstruation. On examination, the discharge may be visible on the labia and fourchette. In the vagina, the discharge (which may be frothy) is milky and adheres to the vaginal walls (see Figure 4.1). There is no inflammation of the vulva or vagina.

DIAGNOSIS

BV can be diagnosed clinically using Amsel's criteria [2]. For a positive diagnosis, three of the following should be present:

- a thin homogenous discharge on examination
- a vaginal pH greater than 4.5
- amine odor on adding 10% potassium hydroxide to the vaginal fluid
- clue cells on microscopy (at least 20% of all epithelial cells covered with bacteria)

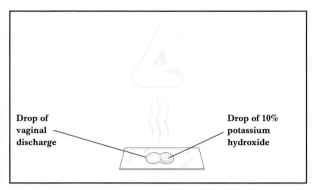

Figure 4.3 The amine whiff test.

The pH should be determined using narrow-range pH paper. The vaginal swab can be touched onto the paper (see Figure 4.2) or the paper can be pressed against the lateral vaginal walls with sponge holders. It is important that cervical secretions are avoided for the pH test because cervical mucus has a pH of 7 and any contamination will give a falsely high reading. To perform the amine test, a loop of vaginal secretions should be mixed with 10% potassium hydroxide on a glass slide. The mixture should be smelt immediately for a transient 'dead fish' odor (see Figure 4.3). A loop of vaginal secretions in a drop of saline should also be examined for clue cells using phase contrast microscopy (wet-mount slide). As a word of warning, if the pH and amine tests are performed within 24 hours of sexual intercourse, in the presence of menstrual blood, or when *T. vaginalis* is present, the pH will be raised and the amine test may be falsely positive.

Recent studies show that a Gram-stained vaginal smear is sensitive and specific for the diagnosis of BV and may be easier to use than Amsel's criteria. To take a vaginal smear for a Gram stain, a swab should be rubbed against the lateral vaginal walls, rolled across a glass side, and allowed to air dry. The slide can then either be Gram stained and interpreted microscopically on-site or be transported to a laboratory for interpretation. This is the easiest and most accurate way of diagnosing BV in clinical settings where on-site microscopy is not available. Culture of vaginal secretions is not a diagnostic test for BV; 30%–50% of women are colonized with *G. vaginalis*, anaerobes, and mycoplasmas as part of their normal vaginal flora.

MANAGEMENT

The UK national guidelines for the management of BV are provided by Hay [3]. Treatment is recommended for all symptomatic women, those undergoing gynecological surgery (including TOP), and pregnant women with a previous preterm birth. Although no treatments are recommended for use during the first trimester of pregnancy, a meta-analysis of metronidazole administration during this period has indicated that it is safe and effective [4,5].

The most effective treatments are oral metronidazole, metronidazole vaginal gel, and clindamycin vaginal cream. Recommended treatment regimens are:

- metronidazole, 400 mg orally, twice daily for 5–7 days
- metronidazole, 2 g orally as a single dose
- metronidazole, 0.75% vaginal gel, 5 g daily for 5 days
- clindamycin, 2% vaginal cream, 5 g daily for 7 days

All of these treatments have a 70%–80% cure rate at 4 weeks. Clindamycin cream may weaken condoms.

As BV is an imbalance of the vaginal bacteria with reduced lactobacilli and a raised vaginal pH, yogurt, acetic acid gel, lactic acid gel, and estrogen creams have all been proposed as treatments. None of these appear to be more effective than placebo [6].

Several randomized placebo-controlled trials have investigated the effect of treatment of the male partner. No reduction in the BV recurrence rate was observed. Therefore, sexual partners do not need to be treated.

RECURRENT INFECTIONS

It should not be assumed that recurrent symptoms mean a recurrence of the infection. It is important to confirm that recurrences are due to BV. The reasons for recurrent BV are not fully understood; it may be due to persistence of BV-associated bacteria following treatment or failure to re-establish normal lactobacilli, and hence the normal pH, following therapy. A rise in the pH results in proliferation of colonizing anaerobes and gardnerella. This explains why BV can recur after menstruation, douching, and sex.

Attempts to restore the vaginal lactobacilli with yogurt vaginally may seem rational but therapeutic trials have shown this to be ineffective. Other vaginal therapies that lower the vaginal pH are ineffective as treatments but they may help to reduce recurrences once BV has been treated and cleared.

The IUD is associated with recurrent BV so, in women with recurrent infection, another form of contraception should be considered. As semen raises the vaginal pH and can therefore facilitate growth of BV-associated bacteria, condoms may help to reduce recurrences.

COMPLICATIONS

There are a number of serious complications associated with BV:

- vaginal cuff cellulitis following hysterectomy
- postpartum endometritis following Cesarean section
- postabortal pelvic inflammatory disease (PID) after surgical TOP
- an increased risk of preterm birth and miscarriage
- a 2- to 3-fold increased risk of contracting human immunodeficiency virus (HIV) in women [7]

These complications are covered in more detail in Chapters 5 and 6.

Candida infections

PREVALENCE RATES

It is estimated that 75% of women have at least one episode of symptomatic candida during their lifetime and 40%–50% will have a further episode. Since clotrimazole became an over-the-counter medication in the US, approximately 13 million treatments have been sold annually. About 20% of asymptomatic women are colonized with candida. Increased rates of colonization (30%–40%) are found during pregnancy and in uncontrolled diabetics [8].

ETIOLOGY

Candida albicans causes 90% of vaginal yeast infections, with *Candida glabrata* and other candida species causing the remaining 10%. There are some recognized predisposing factors, affecting either local or systemic immunity, that encourage candida to become symptomatic. These factors are pregnancy, diabetes, immunosuppression, antimicrobial therapy, and vulval irritation/trauma [9]. However, many women without these predisposing factors develop a vaginal infection. The rarity of candida infections premenarche and postmenopausally suggests a sex hormone dependence. This is also suggested by the characteristic onset of symptoms in the week prior to menstruation in those women with recurrent infections. Although men can be colonized with candida, and many male sexual partners of women with candida are transiently colonized, it is not recognized as an STI. Placebo-controlled studies have not shown a reduction in recurrent infection by treating male partners.

CLINICAL MANIFESTATIONS

Vulval itching is the most common symptom and is present in nearly all symptomatic patients. The typical curdy white vaginal discharge is present in about 50% of

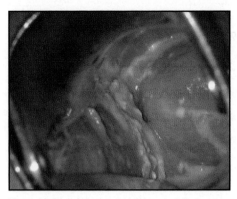

Figure 4.4 Clinical picture of candida vaginal discharge.

symptomatic women but the discharge is frequently minimal. Vulval burning, external dysuria, vaginal soreness, and dyspareunia are also often present. Odor is usually minimal and non-offensive. On examination, vulval erythema and fissuring may be present and can extend to the perianal region. In severe cases, labial edema may occur. There may be typical white plaques adhering to the vaginal walls (see Figure 4.4).

DIAGNOSIS

About 50% of candida infections can be diagnosed by identifying yeast cells and pseudohyphae on a Gram-stained vaginal smear and/or a wet-mount slide. By adding a few drops of 10% potassium hydroxide to the wet-mount specimen, the sensitivity can be improved to 70% as this removes debris and mucus, but it also kills trichomonads. If microscopy is negative but candida infection is suspected, culture should be performed. Sabouraud's medium is widely used and supports the growth of all clinically important yeasts. If culture plates are not available for direct plating, the vaginal swab can be placed in Amies, Stuart's, or similar transport medium. Although vaginal culture is the most sensitive diagnostic method, a positive culture does not necessarily indicate that candida is responsible for the vaginal symptoms because of asymptomatic colonization in about 20% of women. Quantitative cultures have revealed that asymptomatic carriers usually have fewer than 10 colonies per plate. *C. albicans* can be distinguished from non-albicans species by the germ-tube test. Another diagnostic test, though one that is not widely used, is a latex agglutination slide technique (sensitivity of about 80%).

MANAGEMENT

UK guidelines for the management of vulvovaginal candidiasis are provided by Daniels and Forster [9]. There are a number of effective intravaginal and oral antifungal agents available, all with efficacies of 80%–85%. Nystatin is the treatment of choice for *C. glabrata* and other non-albicans species.

Topical treatments:

- clotrimazole, 500 mg as a single pessary
- clotrimazole, a 200 mg pessary for 3 nights
- clotrimazole, a 100 mg pessary for 6 nights
- clotrimazole, 5 g as a single dose of 10% vaginal cream
- econazole*, 150 mg as a single pessary
- econazole*, a 150 mg pessary for 3 nights
- fenticonazole*, 600 mg as a single pessary
- fenticonazole*, a 200 mg pessary for 3 nights
- isoconazole, a 300 mg vaginal tablet for 2 nights
- miconazole*, a 1.2 g single ovule
- miconazole*, a 100 mg pessary for 14 nights
- nystatin, 1 or 2 pessaries (100 000 units) for 14 nights

*damages latex condoms and diaphragms

Oral treatments:

- fluconazole, 150 mg as a single dose
- itraconazole, a 200 mg dose twice for 1 day

Oral therapies should not be used during pregnancy. Sexual partners do not need to be treated unless they also have typical candida symptoms.

RECURRENT CANDIDA

Recurrent candida is defined as at least four mycologically proven symptomatic episodes in 1 year. Some of these women have recognized risk factors but most do not. Occasionally, recurrent candida is caused by the non-albicans species which are resistant to treatment with azoles and triazoles; nystatin is more effective. Without culture and identification of the yeast these resistant types can be missed. In most women, fully sensitive *C. albicans* is responsible for recurrent infections. Longitudinal data, using polymerase chain reaction (PCR) on vaginal swabs and washings, have confirmed that recurrent infection is with the same strain of yeast because of incomplete eradication on treatment [10]. A longer course of topical or oral therapy may prove beneficial.

For women with monthly recurrences, prophylactic pessaries or oral therapies can be used prior to, or immediately after, menses. In placebo-controlled trials, such women have fewer episodes of recurrence while using prophylaxis. Alternatively, episodic treatment can be used at the onset of symptoms. This approach results in more episodes of infection but the total amount of antifungal drugs required (and hence cost) is less.

It is not necessary to stop a low-dose combined oral contraceptive (COC) pill. Oral nystatin and yeast-free diets are ineffective.

COMPLICATIONS
Fortunately, to date, no long-term physical complications from candida infections have been identified. A study of over 13 000 women found no adverse pregnancy outcome [11]. However, women with recurrent candida frequently have psychosexual problems and psychological morbidity.

Trichomonas vaginalis

PREVALENCE RATES
This infection is now relatively rare in the UK and other countries in northern Europe. However, in other parts of the world (Africa and Asia), *T. vaginalis* remains a major cause of vaginal discharge. Prevalence rates of up to 34% have been found in some parts of Africa [12].

ETIOLOGY
T. vaginalis is a protozoa, 10–20 μm in diameter (about the size of a white blood cell). It is sexually transmitted and only infects the urogenital tract. High infection levels are found in the sexual partners of those with a documented infection. Several studies have shown an increased cure rate in women when their sexual partners are treated. *T. vaginalis* is associated with other STIs such as gonorrhea and chlamydia.

Women are the main carriers of the infection. Unlike women, some men may be able to clear the organism. One study found that 70% of men were infected 2 days after sexual intercourse with an infected woman. The infection rate dropped to 33% after 14 days [13].

CLINICAL MANIFESTATIONS
Asymptomatic infections have been reported in 10%–50% of women. This wide variation in range depends upon the selection of the study population; the lowest rates have been reported in women presenting to STI clinics and the highest rates in

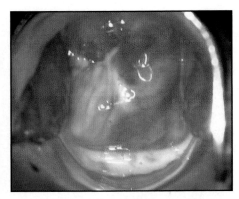

Figure 4.5 Clinical picture of *Trichomonas vaginalis*.

well-women screening programs. Asymptomatic women may become symptomatic, suggesting that changes in the host may contribute to the pathogenic expression. Many women report the initiation or exacerbation of *T. vaginalis* symptoms during, or immediately following, the menstrual period.

A yellow vaginal discharge is the most common symptom in symptomatic women. About 50% also report a malodor due to amine production by anaerobic bacteria (similar to BV). About 25%–50% of women will also have vulval pruritus, which can be severe. External dysuria and dyspareunia may also be present. On examination, 10%–30% of women will have vulval erythema and excoriation. The purulent vaginal discharge may be visible on the vulva prior to speculum examination. The vaginal mucosa is often erythematous. The commonly described, yellow-green, frothy discharge is evident in less than 50% of women; more frequently it has a gray color (see Figure 4.5). The squamous epithelium of the cervix may be inflamed and occasionally has punctate hemorrhages (referred to as the strawberry cervix). Some women with trichomoniasis show no evidence of discharge or inflammation on examination.

DIAGNOSIS

Up to 80% of *T. vaginalis* cases will be detected by microscopy of a wet-mount slide. The trichomonads are best identified by their motility (they are motile because they possess flagella). An increased number of polymorphonuclear leukocytes is usually also observed. At least 20% of women with *T. vaginalis* will not be detected if wet-mount examination alone is used. Culture, usually in a liquid medium, is a more sensitive detection method. The medium is inoculated with a loop of vaginal fluid from the posterior fornix and the culture is incubated at 33–37°C. If *T. vaginalis* culture medium is not available for direct inoculation, a vaginal swab can be placed in Amies, Stuart's, or similar transport medium; however, this may slightly reduce the sensitivity. Various staining methods (acridine orange or fluorescein-labeled monoclonal antibodies) have been used to detect trichomonads on vaginal smears. These staining methods are less sensitive than culture but more sensitive than a wet-mount slide.

Until recently, culture was considered to be the conventional 'gold standard' diagnostic method. A PCR technique for detection of *T. vaginalis* has now been developed with a much better sensitivity rate than culture; however, this technique is still not widely available. In one study using conventional techniques, *T. vaginalis* was detected in 8.6% of women, whereas 15.8% were positive with PCR. Using PCR as the reference, the sensitivity of microscopy was 31% and the sensitivity of culture was 52.8% [14].

T. vaginalis can be observed on Papanicolaou (Pap) smears taken for cervical cytology. The sensitivity may be low so this should not be used as a method of detection. It may also have poor specificity. One study found that 30% of women with *T. vaginalis* reported on a Pap smear had a negative *T. vaginalis* culture [15].

MANAGEMENT
UK guidelines for the management of *T. vaginalis* are provided by Sherrard [16]. Most strains are highly susceptible to metronidazole. A single 2 g dose results in an 80%–85% cure rate. This is increased to 95% with simultaneous treatment of sexual partners.

T. vaginalis infection during pregnancy should be treated as it is associated with an adverse outcome. As with BV, metronidazole is not recommended in the first trimester of pregnancy but, on examination of the literature, it does appear to be safe [4,5].

About 30% of women with *T. vaginalis* will also have either gonorrhea or chlamydia, so a full screen should be performed. Sexual partners should be treated for *T. vaginalis* and screened for other STIs.

RECURRENT INFECTIONS
Recurrent trichomoniasis is usually due to non-compliance with treatment regimes or failure to treat a sexual partner. Most strains of *T. vaginalis* are highly susceptible to metronidazole but resistant strains are occasionally identified. The basis of resistance appears to be aerotolerance. High-dose oral and concurrent intravaginal metronidazole may have a higher efficacy but less than 50% of women will respond. No universally effective alternative treatment is available so referral to a specialist in this field is recommended.

COMPLICATIONS

T. vaginalis in pregnancy is associated with low birth weight and preterm delivery [17]. In a study of the effect of non-ulcerative STIs on the risk of acquiring HIV infection, *T. vaginalis* in women increased the risk, but after adjusting for gonorrhea and chlamydia the adjusted odds ratio (OR) was not significant (OR: 1.9; 95% confidence interval: 0.9–4.1) [18]. Recent studies indicate that there is a definite association between *T. vaginalis* and HIV and that the prevalence of *T. vaginalis* may in part explain the variation in HIV levels between different regions in Africa [12].

Chlamydia trachomatis

PREVALENCE

In the UK, *C. trachomatis* infection affects at least 3%–5% of sexually active women attending general practice. Recent community pilot studies using PCR have found rates of 14% in women under 20 years of age. Therefore, this infection is considered to be a serious public health issue.

ETIOLOGY

C. trachomatis is sexually transmitted in adults. Approximately 60%–70% of sexual partners will also be infected. The primary site of infection in women is the cervix with the urethra also being infected in about 50% of cases. Other sites of infection are the rectum and pharynx. The urethra is the primary infection site in those who have had a hysterectomy.

Many research groups have looked at demographic variables, history, and examination findings in an attempt to identify the best indicators of chlamydial infection. It has consistently been found that an age of less than 25 years is the best predictor of infection. Within this age group, universal screening is the most cost-effective detection strategy as history and examination are not good predictors of infection. Several groups have shown that screening for chlamydia reduces the rate of PID [19]. In 1998, the Chief Medical Officer's (CMO's) Expert Advisory Group on *Chlamydia trachomatis* advised on who should currently be tested for chlamydia and whether chlamydia screening would be cost-effective in the UK [20]. The recommendation was that targeted screening of those under 25 years would be cost-effective, and two pilot studies, in Portsmouth and the Wirral, have been undertaken to look at the feasibility of chlamydia screening in the community. This screening is now being extended to 10 locations with the intention of eventually becoming a national screening programme [21].

The COC pill increases susceptibility to chlamydia infection by increasing the amount of columnar epithelium on the ectocervix. Barrier methods of contraception protect against acquisition.

CLINICAL MANIFESTATIONS

The majority of women (approximately 80%) with chlamydial infection are asymptomatic. If symptoms are present they are usually non-specific, e.g. increased vaginal discharge and dysuria. If the infection has spread beyond the cervix, lower abdominal pain and intermenstrual bleeding may be present. On examination, the cervix may look normal but there may be a mucopurulent cervicitis and/or contact bleeding (see Figures 4.6 and 4.7).

DIAGNOSIS

As *C. trachomatis* is an intracellular bacteria, it can only be grown in cell culture. Therefore, culture is not suitable as a method of diagnosis in most clinical settings. Currently, in the UK, the most commonly used method of diagnosis is enzyme immunoassay (EIA). Unfortunately, some EIA methods have sensitivities of only 60%–70%. To detect chlamydia by EIA it is important that the sites of infection are sampled. Often samples are only taken from the endocervix, but, by also including a urethral sample, the sensitivity can be improved by about 10%. Cellular material must be obtained when taking swabs. For an endocervical specimen, the swab needs to be inserted about 1 cm into the endocervical canal. It should then be rotated vigorously for about 10 seconds before being placed in the EIA kit container. For a urethral specimen, a fine swab should be inserted gently into the urethral opening. It should be rotated gently through about 180 degrees before being placed in the same container as the endocervical sample. As EIA does not rely on culturing the bacterium, urgent transport to the laboratory is not required. Using this method of detection, it is important to recognize that a significant number of infected women may be missed.

Levels of detection can be increased to over 90% by using a DNA amplification test such as PCR or ligase chain reaction on an endocervical swab or first-void urine sample. However, these tests are more expensive than EIA. First-void urine can be used instead of the urethral sample because DNA amplification is more sensitive than EIA and culture. The first 5–10 mL of urine should be collected in a sterile container. A mid-stream urine specimen is not suitable. Non-invasive testing such as first-void urine would obviously be the ideal test if chlamydia screening were ever introduced.

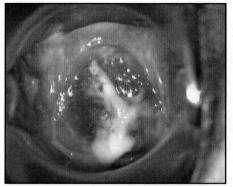
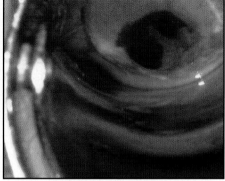

Figure 4.6 Clinical picture of mucopurulent cervicitis.   **Figure 4.7** Clinical picture of contact bleeding of the cervix.

The CMO's Expert Advisory Group on *C. trachomatis* recommended that the following women should be tested for chlamydia [20]:

- women with acute PID
- women with mucopurulent cervicitis
- women with lower abdominal pain
- women with vaginal discharge
- women with postcoital or intermenstrual bleeding
- women requesting TOP

It also recommended that the following women should be considered for testing:

- women seeking infertility treatment
- women undergoing instrumentation of the uterus
- women undergoing IUD insertion
- women undergoing colposcopy

MANAGEMENT

An overview of the management of chlamydia infection is provided by Horner and Caul [22]. Recommended treatments for uncomplicated chlamydia infection are:

- doxycycline, 100 mg twice daily for 1 week
- azithromycin, 1 g orally as a single dose

Both are highly effective with good cure rates. Azithromycin has the convenience of being a single-dose treatment but it is more expensive than doxycycline.

During pregnancy and lactation:

- erythromycin, 500 mg twice daily for 14 days is recommended, although this is not as effective and is tolerated less well than the above treatments
- the safety of azithromycin during pregnancy and in lactating mothers has not yet been fully assessed but available data indicate that it is effective [23]
- amoxycillin, 500 mg three times a day for 7 days, has been shown to have a similar cure rate to erythromycin, 500 mg four times a day for 7 days, but has a better side-effect profile. However, it should only be prescribed in conjunction with a genitourinary medicine (GUM) or specialist STI service as there are serious concerns that amoxycillin may not truly cure the infection as it can induce latency *in vitro*.

Patients should be told to abstain from sex until they and their partner(s) have completed treatment. Partner notification (contact tracing) is an essential part of the management to prevent reinfection. If this cannot be organized by you then the patient should be referred to a GUM or specialist STI service.

All patients should have a follow-up assessment to ensure that:
- medication has been completed
- there has been sexual abstinence
- the partner(s) has been treated

A test for cure following an uncomplicated infection is not necessary if all of the above have been followed, unless erythromycin has been prescribed (because of its low cure rate). However, a test for cure after completion of therapy is recommended for all pregnant women because of the potential for vertical transmission and because erythromycin is usually the therapy used. If a DNA amplification test is used to detect chlamydia, the repeat swab should be delayed until 3 weeks after the treatment has been completed to avoid false positive results.

RECURRENT INFECTIONS
Recurrent infections are usually due to non-compliance with treatment (in which case azithromycin is the treatment of choice) or reinfection from an untreated partner. Adequate contact tracing and advice about sexual abstinence until completion of treatment will be needed.

COMPLICATIONS

C. trachomatis can cause a number of serious complications. It can spread beyond the urethra and cervix and cause Skene's and Bartholin's gland abscesses, endometritis, salpingitis, and perihepatitis. Consequently, tubal pregnancies and tubal infertility can occur. At least 8%–10% of women with chlamydia develop a symptomatic ascending infection but the overall figure is higher because, in some women, the upper genital tract infection is asymptomatic. The risk of an ascending infection is increased with instrumentation such as surgical TOP and IUD insertion. To reduce the rate of postabortal PID, The Royal College of Obstetricians and Gynaecologists of London has recommended that women undergoing surgical TOP should either be tested and treated prior to the termination or be given antibiotics to treat a potential chlamydial infection following it [24]. During pregnancy, chlamydia can cause miscarriage, preterm birth, postpartum infection, and neonatal infection. These complications are covered more fully in Chapters 5 and 6. Conjunctivitis can occur if infected secretions are introduced into the eye. Reactive arthritis (Reiter's syndrome) can occur in genetically susceptible individuals. Chlamydia also increases a woman's risk of acquiring HIV infection by 3- to 4-fold [18] and recent studies have shown a link with cervical cancer [25].

Gonorrhea

PREVALENCE RATES

Neisseria gonorrhoeae infections are much less common than chlamydial infections but there has been a rise in the number of cases over the past few years, particularly in women between 15–19 years old. The Department of Health has set a target of a 25% reduction in gonorrhea infections by 2007, according to The National Strategy for Sexual Health and HIV [21].

ETIOLOGY

In adults, gonorrhea is a sexually transmitted bacterial infection caused by *N. gonorrhoeae*. Between 60%–80% of sexual partners will also be infected. The sites of infection in females are the urethra, cervix, rectum, and pharynx. The primary site of infection in women is the cervix but the urethra is also infected in 70%–90% of cases. As with *C. trachomatis* infections, the urethra becomes the primary infection site in women who have had a hysterectomy. The COC pill may increase susceptibility to gonorrhea by increasing the amount of columnar epithelium on the ectocervix. Barrier contraception methods protect against acquisition.

CLINICAL MANIFESTATIONS

Gonorrhea in women is often asymptomatic (50% of cases). When present, the most common symptoms include increased vaginal discharge, dysuria, and postcoital bleeding. If the infection has spread beyond the cervix, lower abdominal pain and intermenstrual bleeding may also be present. On examination, the cervix may look normal but there may be a purulent or mucopurulent cervicitis and/or contact bleeding (see Figures 4.6 and 4.7). Purulent exudate may occasionally be expressed from the urethra, periurethra, and Bartholin's gland duct.

DIAGNOSIS

Culture of *N. gonorrhoeae* remains the 'gold standard' method of diagnosis. It is inexpensive, sensitive, and available in all laboratories. It also allows antibiotic sensitivity testing. As the main sites of infection are the urethra and endocervix, swabs should be taken from these areas. Specimens should be taken as described for chlamydia detection. If an endocervical swab alone is taken, only 85% of cases of infection will be detected. It is therefore advisable to take urethral samples also. If available, microscopy of a Gram-stained smear of the urethral and cervical swabs can be performed. The Gram-negative diplococci, observed within the polymorphonuclear leukocytes, can be identified on up to 50% of slides. Genital samples should be directly inoculated if selective gonococcal culture medium and facilities for incubation are available. If not available, specimens can be placed in Amies, Stuart's, or similar transport medium. They should be transported to the laboratory as quickly as possible. Studies have shown that there is no reduction in sensitivity before 2 hours but by 24 hours there is a severe decline in viable *N. gonorrhoeae*. Although a high vaginal swab may detect gonorrhea, the sensitivity is poor (only 60%–70%) because *N. gonorrhoeae* is a cervical, not a vaginal, pathogen.

MANAGEMENT

An overview of the management of gonorrhea in adults is provided by Bignell [26]. These UK national guidelines for the management of gonorrhea recommend the referral of patients to a GUM or specialist STI service. Treatments for uncomplicated gonorrhea are:

- ciprofloxacin, 500 mg as a single oral dose
- ofloxacin, 400 mg as a single oral dose
- 3 g of ampicillin and 1 g of probenecid as a single oral dose (if there is a low regional prevalence of penicillin resistance)

Treatment during pregnancy and lactation:

- ceftriaxone, 250 mg intramuscular (IM) as a single dose
- cefotaxime, 500 mg IM as a single dose
- 3 g of ampicillin and 1 g of probenecid (if there is a low regional prevalence of penicillin resistance)

Females with gonorrhea should also be tested and/or treated for chlamydia infection as about 40% will be coinfected with *C. trachomatis*. Patients should be told to abstain from sex until they and their partner(s) have completed treatment. To prevent reinfection, partner notification (contact tracing) is an essential part of management. If this cannot be organized by you then the patient should be referred to a GUM or specialist STI service.

All patients should be seen after treatment to check that medication has been completed, that there has been sexual abstinence, and that the partner(s) has been treated. It is normal practice to repeat the swabs to check that the infection has cleared.

RECURRENT INFECTIONS
Treatment failure due to antibiotic resistance may result in recurrent infections. A second treatment based on the antibiotic sensitivities of the isolate should be given. Treatment failure due to non-compliance is rare with gonorrhea as therapies take the form of a single dose. Recurrent infection may also be due to reinfection from an untreated partner. Adequate contact tracing and advice about sexual abstinence until completion of treatment is essential.

COMPLICATIONS
N. gonorrhoeae can cause a number of serious complications. It can cause Skene's and Bartholin's gland abscesses (see Figure 4.8). Infection can spread to the upper genital tract causing endometritis, salpingitis, and perihepatitis, resulting in tubal pregnancies and tubal infertility. About 10%–20% of women with an acute gonococcal infection will develop salpingitis [27]. The risk of an ascending infection is increased with instrumentation such as surgical TOP and IUD insertion. During pregnancy, gonorrhea can cause miscarriage, preterm birth, postpartum infection, and neonatal infection. These complications are covered more fully in Chapters 5 and 6. Gonococcal conjunctivitis can occasionally occur in adults. Gonococcal septicemia can occur, although it is rare, presenting as an acute arthritis/dermatitis syndrome

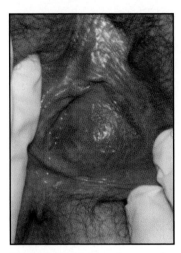

Figure 4.8 Clinical picture of gonococcal
Bartholin's gland abscess.

(disseminated gonococcal infection). Gonorrhea also increases a woman's risk of contracting HIV by 4- to 5-fold [18].

References

1. Wawer MJ, Sewankambo NK, Serwadda D et al. Control of sexually transmitted diseases for AIDS prevention in Uganda: a randomised community trial. Rakai Project Study Group. *Lancet* 1999;353:525–35.

2. Amsel R, Totten PA, Spiegel CA et al. Nonspecific vaginitis. Diagnostic criteria and microbial and epidemiological associations. *Am J Med* 1983;74:14–22.

3. Hay P. National guideline for the management of bacterial vaginosis. *Sex Transm Infect* 1999;75(Suppl. 1):S16–8.

4. Burtin P, Taddio A, Ariburnu O et al. Safety of metronidazole in pregnancy: a meta-analysis. *Am J Obstet Gynecol* 1995;172:525–9.

5. Caro-Paton T, Carvajal A, Martin de Diego I et al. Is metronidazole teratogenic? A meta-analysis. *Br J Clin Pharmacol* 1997;44:179–82.

6. Hillier S, Arko R. Vaginal infections. In: Morse SA, Moreland AA, Holmes KK, editors. *Atlas of sexually transmitted diseases and AIDS*. 2nd edition. London: Mosby-Wolfe, 1996.

7. Taha TE, Hoover DR, Dallabetta GA et al. Bacterial vaginosis and disturbances of vaginal flora: association with increased acquisition of HIV. *AIDS* 1998;12:1699–706.

8. Bland PB. Experimental vaginal and cutaneous moniliasis: clinical and laboratory studies of certain monilias associated with vaginal, oral and cutaneous thrush. *Arch Dermatol Syphil* 1937;36:760.

9. Daniels D, Forster G. National guideline for the management of vulvovaginal candidiasis. *Sex Transm Infect* 1999;75(Suppl. 1):S19–20.

10. El-Din SS, Reynolds MT, Ashbee HR et al. An investigation into the pathogenesis of vulvo-vaginal candidosis. *Sex Transm Infect* 2001;77:179–83.

11. Cotch MF, Hillier SL, Gibbs RS et al. Epidemiology and outcomes associated with moderate to heavy candida colonisation during pregnancy. *Am J Obstet Gynecol* 1998;178:374–80.

12. Buve A, Weiss HA, Laga M et al. The epidemiology of trichomoniasis in women in four African cities. *AIDS* 2001;15(Suppl. 4):S89–96.

13. Weston TE, Nicol CS. Natural history of trichomonal infection in males. *Br J Vener Dis* 1963;39:251–7.

14. Paterson BA, Tabrizi SN, Garland SM et al. The tampon test for trichomoniasis: a comparison between conventional methods and a polymerase chain reaction for *Trichomonas vaginalis* in women. *Sex Transm Infect* 1998;74:136–9.

15. Waghorn DJ, Tucker PK, Chia Y et al. Collaborative approach to improve the detection and management of trichomoniasis in a low prevalence district. *Int J STD AIDS* 1998;9:164–7.

16. Sherrard J. National guideline for the management of *Trichomonas vaginalis*. *Sex Transm Infect* 1999;75 (Suppl. 1):S21–3.

17. Cotch MF, Pastorek JG, Nugent RP et al. *Trichomonas vaginalis* associated with low birth weight and preterm delivery. *Sex Transm Dis* 1997;24:353–60.

18. Laga M, Manoka A, Kivuvu M et al. Non-ulcerative sexually transmitted diseases as risk factors for HIV-1 transmission in women: results from a cohort study. *AIDS* 1993;7:95–102.

19. Scholes D, Stergachis A, Heidrich FE et al. Prevention of pelvic inflammatory disease by screening for cervical chlamydial infection. *N Engl J Med* 1996;334:1362–6.

20. Metters JS, editor. *Chlamydia trachomatis*. Summary and conclusions of the CMO's Expert Advisory Group. London: Department of Health, 1998.

21. The National Strategy for Sexual Health and HIV. Implementation action plan. London: Department of Health, 2002. Available at: URL: http://www.doh.gov.uk/sexualhealthandhiv/pdfs/77007better presersex.pdf

22. Horner PJ, Caul EO. Management of *Chlamydia trachomatis* genital tract infection. *Sex Transm Infect* 1999;75 (Suppl. 1):S4–8.

23. Miller JM Jr. Efficacy and tolerance of single-dose azithromycin for treatment of chlamydial cervicitis during pregnancy. *Infect Dis Obstet Gynecol* 1995;3:189–92.

24. Templeton A, editor. *The prevention of pelvic infection*. London: RCOG Press, 1996.

25. Koskela P, Anttila T, Bjorge T et al. *Chlamydia trachomatis* infection as a risk factor for invasive cervical cancer. *Int J Cancer* 2000;85:35–9.

26. Bignell C. Management of gonorrhoea in adults. *Sex Transm Infect* 1999;75(Suppl. 1):S13–5.

27. Holmes KK, Eschenbach DA, Knapp JS. Salpingitis: overview of etiology and epidemiology. *Am J Obstet Gynecol* 1980;138:893–900.

chapter 5

Upper genital tract complications
Janet Wilson

Several vaginal and cervical pathogens can ascend the genital tract into the uterus, Fallopian tubes, and peritoneal cavity. The symptoms caused by these pathogens depend upon the level of spread of the infection.

Postcoital bleeding

Postcoital bleeding is often the result of a cervical infection. The two major causal organisms are *Chlamydia trachomatis* and *Neisseria gonorrhoeae*, which affect the endocervix. Cervical condylomata, caused by human papillomavirus (HPV), and cervical ulcers, caused by herpes simplex virus (HSV), can also result in postcoital bleeding. Even though it is a vaginal pathogen, *Trichomonas vaginalis* may occasionally be a cause because the squamous epithelium of the vagina extends onto the ectocervix. The diagnosis and management of these infections are covered in Chapters 3 and 4.

Intermenstrual bleeding

C. trachomatis, *N. gonorrhoeae*, and organisms associated with bacterial vaginosis (BV) can spread to the uterus causing endometritis [1]. Clinically, this presents as irregular or intermenstrual bleeding. Plasma cell endometritis can be detected histologically using an endometrial biopsy. The causal organisms can be isolated from the endometrium, confirming their role in the infection. Chlamydia is a recognized cause of intermenstrual bleeding in combined oral contraceptive (COC) pill users, probably because there is an increased incidence of chlamydia [2] and an increased risk of unrecognized endometritis in these individuals [3].

Pelvic inflammatory disease

Pelvic inflammatory disease (PID) occurs when an infection ascends from the cervix or vagina to the pelvic organs. Conditions that may result from PID include:

- endometritis
- salpingitis
- a tubo-ovarian abscess
- pelvic peritonitis

PREVALENCE RATES

Due to the high incidence of asymptomatic PID – approximately two thirds of cases remain unrecognized [4] – the actual prevalence in the population is unclear. It is the most common gynecological hospital admission in the US, accounting for 49 of every 10 000 hospital discharges [5]. Sexually transmitted infection (STI) clinics in the UK have reported a doubling in the number of cases of chlamydial PID between 1995 and 1999 [6]. The incidence was shown to be highest in women under 25 years of age [6].

ETIOLOGY

The main causal agents are *C. trachomatis* and *N. gonorrhoeae,* but bacteria normally colonizing the vagina and cervix may also play a role. Isolates from the upper genital tract are usually polymicrobial and include *Mycoplasma hominis* and anaerobes. In 1995, a UK-based study reported that 45% of PID cases were attributable to chlamydia and 14% to gonorrhea [7]. Studies from the US have reported higher rates of PID attributed to gonorrhea (40%–50%), consistent with the higher incidence of gonorrhea in the US in comparison to western Europe. It is unclear whether the endogenous bacteria of the lower genital tract are independent risk factors in the pathogenesis of PID or secondary infections following initial damage by *C. trachomatis* and *N. gonorrhoeae*. BV has been implicated as a risk factor for PID, and BV-associated bacteria appear to facilitate the spread of *C. trachomatis* and *N. gonorrhoeae* to the upper genital tract. However, no bacterial cause is identified in a significant proportion of women with PID (identified at laparoscopy) [7].

The risk of an ascending infection is increased with instrumentation such as surgical termination of pregnancy (TOP), hysterosalpingography, and intrauterine device (IUD) insertion. PID is also more common in women who douche [8]. The onset of symptoms is more likely in the first part of the menstrual cycle, suggesting ascent into the upper genital tract after loss of the cervical mucus barrier during menstruation.

The IUD has been associated with an increased risk of PID within the first month after insertion, and prior IUD usage increases the risk of tubal infertility and ectopic pregnancy, suggesting increased rates of PID in IUD users. However, recent reviews have shown that the PID rate is similar in women with asymptomatic gonorrhea or chlamydia, with or without an IUD. Furthermore, using an IUD does not affect tubal fertility [9]. When compared with non-hormonal IUDs, the progesterone implanted intrauterine system protects against salpingitis [10].

As the use of COC reduces the symptoms of upper genital tract infection, it appears to protect against severe PID requiring hospitalization. This may not be a true protection against PID, but rather simply a reduction in symptoms.

CLINICAL MANIFESTATIONS

The clinical presentations are variable, ranging from asymptomatic to very severe. Women with chlamydial PID generally have a clinically milder disease than women with gonococcal PID. Common symptoms of PID include:

- lower abdominal pain (the most common symptom)
- increased vaginal discharge
- irregular bleeding
- deep dyspareunia
- dysuria (occasionally)

On bimanual examination, adnexal and cervical motion tenderness are the most frequently found signs, but pyrexia and a palpable adnexal mass may also be present. A mucopurulent discharge from the cervix with contact bleeding is indicative of cervicitis (see Chapter 4, Figures 4.6 and 4.7). The correlation of clinical and laboratory findings with findings at laparoscopy is provided in Table 5.1 [11].

DIAGNOSIS

There are no symptoms, signs, or laboratory tests that are diagnostic of PID. Laparoscopy, with microbiological specimens from the upper and lower genital tract, is considered the 'gold standard' for diagnosis. However, in practice, diagnosis is often made clinically on the basis of lower abdominal pain, increased vaginal discharge, cervical motion, and adnexal tenderness on bimanual examination. Swabs are only taken from the lower genital tract. Clinical diagnosis has advantages over laparoscopic diagnosis, being quicker, cheaper, and non-invasive, but it is less accurate with a specificity of only 60%–70% [11].

A study from Sweden, comparing a clinical diagnosis with a laparoscopic diagnosis of PID in over 900 women, showed that clinical diagnosis is only accurate 60% of the time (see Table 5.1) [11]. Non-specific tests for inflammation may be carried out such as measuring the erythrocyte sedimentation rate (ESR), a white cell count, or

Clinical/laboratory abnormalities	Laparoscopic diagnosis salpingitis (%)	Laparoscopic diagnosis normal or other (%)	% of women with salpingitis presenting with symptoms or signs
Lower abdominal pain, LGTI, and cervical motion tenderness	61%	39%	16%
Lower abdominal pain, LGTI, cervical motion tenderness plus at least one of: ESR ≥ 15 mm/hour; temperature >38°C; a palpable adnexal mass			
Plus ONE	78%	22%	28%
Plus TWO	90%	10%	39%
Plus all THREE	96%	4%	17%

Table 5.1 The correlation between a clinical diagnosis of PID and findings on laparoscopy [11]. ESR: erythrocyte sedimentation rate; LGTI: lower genital tract infection, defined as the presence of inflammatory cells outnumbering other cellular elements (epithelial cells) on wet-mount examination of vaginal fluid.

acute phase reactants. Since PID arises from a lower genital tract infection, a wet-mount or Gram-stained slide of vaginal fluid should show either bacterial vaginosis or inflammatory cells outnumbering epithelial cells. The absence of this diagnostic characteristic gives a relatively high negative predictive value for PID. In the Swedish study referred to in Table 5.1, none of the women with laparoscopic-verified PID had normal vaginal wet-mount slides [11]. The specificity of the clinical diagnosis can be improved to 96% if three further signs – fever, a raised ESR, and a palpable adnexal mass – are all present. However, this improvement in specificity is to the detriment of the sensitivity, with only 17% of all cases of PID being detected [11]. In view of the serious long-term complications from PID it is more appropriate to use the most sensitive method of diagnosis rather than the most specific. A meta-analysis of PID diagnosis has revealed that adnexal tenderness has a sensitivity of 95% but a specificity of only 74% and a palpable adnexal mass has a sensitivity of 48% but a specificity of 75% [12]. Clinical symptoms and signs do not accurately predict the extent of tubal disease at laparoscopy.

Even laparoscopy is not perfect: the interpretation of findings is subjective, and the technique may not always be immediately available in clinical practice. Endometrial biopsies are easy to obtain and demonstration of histological endometritis has a sensitivity of 89% [13]. The application of non-invasive imaging tests such as color Doppler ultrasound and magnetic resonance imaging for PID diagnosis is being evaluated.

A pregnancy test should be performed on all women suspected of having PID to exclude ectopic pregnancy—a life-threatening differential diagnosis.

MANAGEMENT

Overviews of the management of PID are provided by Ross [14] and Templeton [15]. The patient should be admitted if there is diagnostic uncertainty, failure with oral therapy, or severe symptoms or signs. As prompt diagnosis and appropriate treatment reduce the likelihood of tubal damage [16], empirical treatment should be initiated before microbiology results are known. The antibiotic regimen used should cover the main bacterial causes and take into account local prevalence data and sensitivity patterns. Intravenous (IV) therapy is recommended for women with severe clinical disease. IV treatment should be continued until 24 hours after clinical improvement and then oral therapy should be used. Recommended therapeutic regimens are:

- cefoxitin, 2 g IV three times daily, plus doxycycline, 100 mg (IV or oral) twice daily, plus metronidazole, 400 mg (IV or oral) twice daily, for 14 days

- ofloxacin, 400 mg (IV or oral) twice daily, plus metronidazole 400 mg (IV or oral), for 14 days

- ceftriaxone, 250 mg intramuscular (IM) single dose, or cefoxitin, 2 g IM single dose, with probenecid, 1 g single oral dose, plus doxycycline, 100 mg (IV or oral) twice daily, plus metronidazole, 400 mg (IV or oral) twice daily, for 14 days

Patients should be prescribed appropriate analgesia and be advised to abstain from sex until they and their partner(s) have completed treatment. To prevent reinfection, partner notification (contact tracing) is an essential part of management. If this cannot be organized by you then the patient should be referred to a genitourinary medicine or a specialist STI service.

Review after 2–3 days is recommended for those with moderate or severe clinical findings to check that their condition is starting to improve. If there is no response to treatment, then further investigation, IV therapy and/or surgical intervention are required.

Follow-up after completion of treatment should be arranged to check:

- the clinical response
- that the course of medication has been completed
- that there has been sexual abstinence
- that the partner(s) has been treated

Repeat testing for initially positive infections is recommended. If the method used to detect chlamydia is a DNA amplification test, the repeat swab should be delayed until 3 weeks after treatment has been completed to avoid false positive results.

The Royal College of Obstetricians and Gynaecologists has recommended that [15]:

- all women suspected of having PID should have appropriate testing for chlamydia and gonorrhea
- amplification tests (polymerase chain reaction or ligase chain reaction) should ideally be used for chlamydia detection
- antibiotics administered should cover chlamydia and gonorrhea infections and also infections by anaerobes
- the sexual partner(s) should be contact traced and given empirical treatment

COMPLICATIONS

The complications from PID are:

- tubal infertility [17]   10%–12% of cases after one episode

  20%–30% of cases after two episodes

  50%–60% of cases after three or more episodes
- ectopic pregnancy [18]   6- to 10-fold increased risk
- chronic pain   18% of cases
- hysterectomy [18]   8-fold increased risk

The number of episodes of PID, and the severity of the infection in a woman who has experienced only one episode, significantly affect the rate of tubal infertility. Prompt diagnosis and the correct treatment reduce the likelihood of tubal damage. In women with a chlamydial infection who have delayed treatment, there is a 3-fold increased risk of impaired fertility compared to women who start treatment within 3 days of symptom appearance [16].

With gonococcal infections, tubal damage is caused by an acute neutrophilic inflammatory response. With chlamydial infections, tubal damage results from stimulation of a cell-mediated lymphocytic response and, possibly, a delayed-type hypersensitivity response. Tubal inflammation can be very rapid, within hours for gonorrhea and within days for chlamydia. Tubal scarring occurs as the dead epithelial cells are replaced by fibroblasts, leading to deciliation or occlusion. Scarring begins within days of infection.

In the study from Sweden [11], the ectopic pregnancy rate was 1.3% in control women compared to 7.8% in those with salpingitis. The risk of ectopic pregnancy was shown to increase with increasing episodes and severity of PID.

The number of episodes of PID is related to the incidence of abdominal or pelvic pain for longer than 6 months (either continuous pain or repeated episodes of pain); this occurs in 11.8% of cases with one episode, 30% of cases with two episodes, and 66.7% of cases with three or more episodes of PID. Pain correlates with the extent of pelvic adhesions. Women with a past history of PID are 5–10 times more likely to need hospital admission and hysterectomy than control women [18].

In 5%–15% of women with salpingitis, the infection can spread from the pelvis to the liver capsule causing perihepatitis (Fitz-Hugh–Curtis syndrome). With this condition, the liver parenchyma is normal but 'violin string' adhesions form between the liver capsule and the adjacent parietal peritoneum under the ribs.

Repeated infections occur in about one third of women because of:
- inadequate treatment leading to relapse
- reinfection from an untreated partner
- postinfection damage to tubes
- further acquisition of STIs

To preserve fertility, prevention of further infections is important. Studies in animal models have shown that a single episode of *C. trachomatis* induced salpingitis may often be self-limiting, whereas repeated infections, even of the cervix, eventually produce severe tubal scarring [19]. The immunity acquired during a chlamydial infection in some individuals might therefore cause delayed hypersensitivity reactions during prolonged infections or reinfections. Screening and treating asymptomatic cervical chlamydia infection can reduce the rate of PID [20,21].

References

1. Korn AP, Hessol NA, Padian NS et al. Risk factors for plasma cell endometritis among women with cervical *Neisseria gonorrhoeae*, cervical *Chlamydia trachomatis*, or bacterial vaginosis. *Am J Obstet Gynecol* 1998;178:987–90.

2. Krettek JE, Arkin SI, Chaisilwattana P et al. *Chlamydia trachomatis* in patients who used oral contraceptives and had intermenstrual spotting. *Obstet Gynecol* 1993;81:728–31.

3. Ness RB, Keder LM, Soper DE et al. Oral contraception and the recognition of endometritis. *Am J Obstet Gynecol* 1997;176:580–5.

4. Sellors JW, Mahony JB, Chernesky MA et al. Tubal factor infertility: an association with prior chlamydial infection and asymptomatic salpingitis. *Fertil Steril* 1988;49:451–7.

5. Velebil P, Wingo PA, Xia Z et al. Rate of hospitalization for gynecologic disorders among reproductive-age women in the United States. *Obstet Gynecol* 1995;86:764–9.

6. PHLS, DHSS&PS and the Scottish ISD(D)5 Collaborative Group. Trends in sexually transmitted infections in the United Kingdom, 1990–99. London: Public Health Laboratory Service, 2000.

7. Bevan CD, Johal BJ, Mumtaz G et al. Clinical, laparoscopic and microbiological findings in acute salpingitis: report on a United Kingdom cohort. *Br J Obstet Gynaecol* 1995;102:407–14.

8. Wolner-Hanssen P, Eschenbach DA, Paavonen J et al. Association between vaginal douching and acute pelvic inflammatory disease. *JAMA* 1990;263:1936–41.

9. Grimes DA. Intrauterine device and upper genital tract infection. *Lancet* 2000;356:1013–9.

10. Luukkainen T, Toivonen J. Levonorgestrel-releasing IUD as a method of contraception with therapeutic properties. *Contraception* 1995;52:269–76.

11. Jacobson L, Westrom L. Objectivized diagnosis of pelvic inflammatory disease. *Am J Obstet Gynecol* 1969;105:1088–98.

12. Kahn JG, Walker CK, Washington AE et al. Diagnosing pelvic inflammatory disease. A comprehensive analysis and considerations for developing a new model. *JAMA* 1991;266:2594–604.

13. Paavonen J, Aine R, Teisala K et al. Comparison of endometrial biopsy and peritoneal fluid cytologic testing with laparoscopy in the diagnosis of acute pelvic inflammatory disease. *Am J Obstet Gynecol* 1985;151:645–50.

14. Ross JD. National Guideline for the management of pelvic infection and perihepatitis. *Sex Transm Infect* 1999;75(Suppl. 1):S54–6.

15. Templeton A, editor. *The prevention of pelvic infection*. London: RCOG Press, 1996.

16. Hillis SD, Joesoef R, Marchbanks PA et al. Delayed care of pelvic inflammatory diseases as a risk factor for impaired fertility. *Am J Obstet Gynecol* 1993;168:1503–9.

17. Westrom L, Joesoef R, Reynolds G et al. Pelvic inflammatory disease and fertility. A cohort study of 1844 women with laparoscopically verified disease and 657 control women with normal laparoscopic results. *Sex Transm Dis* 1992;19:185–92.

18. Buchan H, Vessey M, Goldacre M et al. Morbidity following pelvic inflammatory disease. *Br J Obstet Gynaecol* 1993;100:558–62.

19. Patton DL, Wolner-Hanssen P, Cosgrove SJ et al. The effects of *Chlamydia trachomatis* on the female reproductive tract of *Macaca nemestrina* after a single tubal challenge following repeated cervical inoculations. *Obstet Gynecol* 1990;76:643–50.

20. Scholes D, Stergachis A, Heidrich FE et al. Prevention of pelvic inflammatory disease by screening for cervical chlamydial infection. *N Engl J Med* 1996;334:1362–6.

21. Kamwendo F, Forslin L, Bodin L et al. Programmes to reduce pelvic inflammatory disease – the Swedish experience. *Lancet* 1998;351(Suppl. 3):25–8.

chapter 6

Complications of infections in pregnancy and infants

Janet Wilson

Chlamydia trachomatis

Chlamydia trachomatis has been found in 1%–12% of pregnant women attending antenatal clinics and in 7%–12% of women requesting termination of pregnancy (TOP) [1]. It is a well described cause of postabortal pelvic inflammatory disease (PID), with up to 60% of postabortal PID cases being attributable to chlamydial infections. In an attempt to reduce this rate, the Royal College of Obstetricians and Gynaecologists of London has recommended that women undergoing surgical TOP should either be tested and treated for chlamydia infection prior to the termination or be given antibiotics to cover the infection following the procedure [2]. Administering antibiotics postoperatively has been shown to be a more cost-effective approach in the short term but there are concerns about the long-term risks. If prophylactic antibiotics are given at the time of TOP, iatrogenic ascending infection is reduced but infected women are not identified so no attempt can be made to treat their partners. Consequently, these women are likely to become reinfected, with a subsequent risk of PID in the future.

In one study, *C. trachomatis* was isolated from four out of 22 first-trimester abortuses, although no cohort study has ever shown a definite link with miscarriage. Chlamydia can cause tubal infertility and if tubal blockage is incomplete there is an increased risk of future ectopic pregnancy. Women with tubal pregnancies have been shown to have significantly higher rates of *C. trachomatis* antibodies than women with intrauterine pregnancies. Between 33%–59% of ectopic pregnancies have also been attributed to chlamydial infection.

PID (in the absence of any surgical intervention) in pregnancy is rare (when compared to the situation in non-pregnant women). This is probably because, after 12 weeks' gestation, the chorion attaches to the endometrial decidua, obliterating the intrauterine cavity. Therefore, after this period, the route for ascending intraluminal spread is obstructed and the chorioamnion probably becomes the site of ascending infection. A large prospective study has shown that women with *C. trachomatis* at

24 weeks' gestation were 2–3 times more likely to have a preterm birth than uninfected women [3].

Chlamydial infection in neonates is transmitted via perinatal transmission. The vertical transmission rate is 50%–70% [4]. Infection can occur in the conjunctiva, nasopharynx, rectum, and vagina. The most frequent clinical presentation is conjunctivitis, with the most frequent site of infection being the nasopharynx. In chlamydia infection cases presenting after the neonatal period but before the age of 3 years, vertical transmission is the most likely route of infection but sexual abuse will need to be considered.

Conjunctivitis usually presents 5–12 days after birth, most frequently between day 7 and day 8. The clinical manifestations can range from asymptomatic to severe purulent conjunctivitis; the discharge is usually mucopurulent. About one third of infants with a nasopharyngeal infection develop pneumonia. This usually presents between the ages of 4–12 weeks, but occasionally may present as early as 2 weeks. No cases have been reported in babies more than 4 months old. The infection may be asymptomatic and, if untreated, may persist in the nasopharynx for up to 3 years, and in the rectum and vagina for at least 1 year [5].

Microbiological testing is essential for the differentiation of the causes of neonatal conjunctivitis. The Chief Medical Officer's Expert Advisory Group on *Chlamydia trachomatis* recommends testing of all infants with ophthalmia neonatorum or neonatal pneumonia [1].

Culture from the conjunctiva is the 'gold standard' test for chlamydia but access to this in the clinical setting may be difficult. Polymerase chain reaction (PCR) and some enzyme immunoassays (EIAs) have been shown to be equivalent to culture of conjunctival specimens. EIAs do not perform well on nasopharyngeal specimens but PCR is as good as a culture test. EIA should not be used to evaluate rectal or vaginal specimens.

As neonatal chlamydial infection is usually at several sites, topical eye treatment is not adequate therapy for conjunctivitis. Systemic treatment is required, which should consist of oral erythromycin, 50 mg/kg/day, divided into four daily doses for 2 weeks. The cure rate from this is less than 90%, so repeat tests should be performed after treatment. If the infection is still present a further course of treatment should be administered.

Chlamydial infection in female adults is frequently asymptomatic. Infection in the infant may be the first presentation of disease in the mother. The mother must be examined, tested, and treated.

Gonorrhea

Gonorrhea infection has been shown to result in a 3-fold increase in the risk of postabortal endometritis [6]. The effects of gonococcal infection in early pregnancy have not been well studied but early infection can cause septic abortion. As with chlamydia, gonorrhea can cause tubal infertility so may predispose to future ectopic pregnancies. Acute salpingitis can occur early in pregnancy but is rare. The risk of disseminated gonococcal infection is increased in pregnancy.

Prospective studies of gonorrhea in pregnancy have shown a 3- to 6-fold increased risk of preterm birth and low birth weight [7]. A postpartum upper genital tract infection has been reported in 47% of women with intrapartum gonorrhea.

Neonatal gonococcal infections are transmitted via prenatal or perinatal contact with infected amniotic fluid or an infected birth canal. Infection may occur in the conjunctiva, oropharynx, urethra, vagina, and rectum. The most frequent clinical presentation is conjunctivitis. The rate of gonococcal ophthalmia in infants born to women with untreated gonorrhea is approximately 30% [8]. Pharyngeal infection will also be present in one third of those with conjunctivitis. The onset of the ophthalmia neonatorum is typically 2–5 days after birth but it can develop later. The infant develops a profuse, purulent discharge, with edema of the eyelids. If untreated, corneal ulceration, scarring and, occasionally, perforation can occur. There may also be a systemic infection with the most commonly recognized complication being septic arthritis. Rectal and pharyngeal infections are usually asymptomatic and are often unrecognized. The finding of gonorrhea in children over 1 year old is highly suggestive of sexual abuse.

Culture is the appropriate method of diagnosis for all potential sites of infection. Conjunctival exudates can also be examined microscopically, after being Gram stained for typical Gram-negative intracellular diplococci. However, culture must also be performed.

Topical treatment of the eye is inadequate because of the multiple inoculation sites. Systemic therapy is required. If there is low regional prevalence of penicillin resistance, or if the sensitivity of the organism is known in advance of treatment, a single 50 mg/kg dose of oral ampicillin can be used. Alternatively, ceftriaxone, 25–50 mg/kg (not exceeding 125 mg), intravenous (IV) or intramuscular as a single dose can be used. All infants with gonococcal disease should also be tested and/or treated for chlamydial infection. The infection in the infant may be the first presentation of gonorrhea in the mother. The mother must also be examined, tested, and treated.

Genital warts

During pregnancy, genital warts may rapidly enlarge, especially towards the latter part of gestation, and they may be difficult to clear. They very rarely cause any problems in pregnancy or during birth but there have been isolated case reports of labor being obstructed. During the postnatal period spontaneous regression often occurs.

Genital warts presenting within the first year of life are likely to be perinatally transmitted. The rate of vertical transmission appears to be low [9]. Therefore, there is no justification for Cesarean section (CS) in pregnant women because of genital warts. In infants, the warts occur in the larynx and genital (usually perianal) area. Genital warts presenting after infancy are usually acquired following sexual contact.

Genital herpes

Before 20 weeks' gestation, maternal primary herpes has been associated with spontaneous abortion, but the absolute risk of this is not known. Herpes simplex virus (HSV) acquisition in pregnancy is associated with little other pregnancy morbidity but can cause serious neonatal problems. Oral or IV aciclovir should be considered for treatment of the first episode of genital herpes. Although this drug has not been licensed for use in pregnancy it has been widely used and to date there is no evidence of teratogenicity. Less is known about the safety of valaciclovir and famciclovir.

Over 70% of infants with neonatal HSV infection are born to mothers who lack symptoms or signs of HSV lesions at delivery. The risk of transmission of neonatal herpes to the infant from a woman with primary HSV at the time of delivery is about 40%. In women with past HSV-1 and new HSV-2 the risk of transmission is 20%, and in women with recurrent HSV-2 at the time of delivery the risk is less than 1% [10]. These data suggest that passive neonatal immunity from maternal HSV-2 specific antibodies is protective to the infant. Maternal primary infection, particularly late in pregnancy, may not result in significant passage of maternal antibodies across the placenta to the fetus. Also, the amount of virus shed, and the length of time of shedding, is much greater with primary rather than recurrent infection. The duration of membrane rupture is also a risk factor. Prolonged rupture of membranes (longer than 6 hours) increases the risk of virus acquisition. Fetal scalp monitors can be a site of inoculation and may increase the risk [11]. They should be avoided in women with a history of recurrent HSV. The outcome of neonatal HSV is so devastating that many women have elected to deliver by CS; many have had a CS unnecessarily. Cultures obtained for HSV prior to delivery do not predict neonatal infection [12].

If a primary attack occurs within the 6 weeks immediately before delivery, then CS is recommended to reduce perinatal transmission of the virus. If vaginal delivery is unavoidable, aciclovir treatment of the mother and baby should be considered. Women with primary infection in the first and second trimesters are at high risk of recurrences in the last trimester. Aciclovir, 400 mg given twice daily continuously in the last 4 weeks of pregnancy, may prevent a recurrence at term and therefore may abolish the need for CS [13].

With known recurrent genital herpes, vaginal delivery is appropriate if no lesions are present at the time of birth. In the UK, current practice is CS if there is an active recurrence during labor. However, even with an active lesion, the risk of vertical transmission following vaginal delivery is small and should be set against the risks of CS to the mother [14].

Neonatal herpes can be acquired *in utero*, intrapartum, or postnatally. The mother is the source of the infection for the first two routes, and may also be the source for the third but this infection could come from another contact or even a healthcare worker. Most cases (80%–90%) are acquired intrapartum. The estimated incidence in the UK is 1.65 per 100 000 live births. Higher rates of seven per 100 000 have been reported in the US. Both HSV-1 and HSV-2 can cause neonatal herpes.

Neonatal herpes is almost always symptomatic and frequently fatal. There are three categories of infection:

- localization of the disease to the site of viral entry (usually the skin, eyes, or mouth)
- encephalitis
- disseminated infection involving the brain and multiple other organs

Disseminated infection has the worst prognosis for both morbidity and mortality. Not all infants with disseminated infection develop skin vesicles which can make diagnosis difficult. In the absence of therapy, mortality is 80% and virtually all those who survive have some residual impairment. The mortality rate without treatment for encephalitis is 50%. Death is not usually associated with infection of the skin, eyes, or mouth but 70% of cases will progress to encephalitis or disseminated infection if not treated.

As the signs of neonatal herpes can be non-specific, the diagnosis is often indicated by having a high index of suspicion. A positive maternal HSV culture or history of genital herpes symptoms in either the mother or a sexual partner reinforces the suspicion of neonatal HSV infection. If vesicles are present in the baby, fluid can be sent for electron microscopy examination and culture.

The treatment of choice for neonatal HSV infections is IV aciclovir. The recommended dose is 10 mg/kg IV every 8 hours for 10–14 days. Even after this treatment some infants have relapsed and higher doses and treatment for longer periods of time are being investigated. Following treatment, mortality rates have dropped to 55% for disseminated infections, 18% for encephalitis, and 0% for skin, eye, or mouth infections. Neurological impairment of the survivors is also reduced with treatment [15].

Bacterial vaginosis

Bacterial vaginosis (BV) can cause postabortal PID after surgical TOP. Treatment with metronidazole at the time of termination can reduce this. The Royal College of Obstetricians and Gynaecologists of London has recommended that women undergoing surgical TOP should be given metronidazole to reduce the rate of postabortal PID [2]. BV is an independent risk factor for preterm birth, increasing the risk of premature delivery to between 1.4–7 times normal levels [16]. The premature labor is secondary to an ascending vaginal infection causing chorioamnionitis. As BV is a common infection, it has been estimated that the population attributable risk of premature delivery due to BV in the US is 30%, and this is estimated to cost $1 billion annually [17]. BV also increases the risk of second-trimester miscarriage by 3- to 4-fold [16], and doubles the risk of first-trimester miscarriage [18]. It can cause postpartum endometritis following CS.

Women with a previous preterm birth benefit from treatment of BV in subsequent pregnancies [19]. However, the published randomized placebo-controlled trials in all pregnant women (pregnant women who have or have not had a preterm birth) have not shown any treatment benefit [20], so as yet there is no evidence to support screening all pregnant women for BV.

Although the presence of BV in pregnancy may cause prematurity and low birth weight due to preterm birth, it has no direct effect on the infant.

Trichomoniasis

A study of over 13 000 pregnant women found a 1.3-fold increased risk of low birth weight and preterm delivery in women with trichomoniasis. In one study, 11% of low birth weights in black women, and 1.5% of low birth weights in white women were attributed to trichomoniasis infection [21]. As with BV, other than the effects of prematurity, there are no direct consequences of the infection on the infant.

Syphilis

The most common outcome of early syphilis in pregnancy is miscarriage and stillbirth during the second and early third trimesters. Most transmission to the infant occurs *in utero*. The risk of congenital syphilis is related to the stage of infection in the mother. Transmission rates are extremely high during the first 4 years after acquiring the infection. In women with untreated syphilis of less than 4 years, 41% of infants were born with congenital syphilis, 25% were stillborn and 14% were neonatal deaths. Only 18% were normal full-term infants. In women with untreated late syphilis of over 4 years, only 2% of infants had congenital syphilis [22]. The purpose of antenatal syphilis serology is to detect women with untreated syphilis in pregnancy, as treatment of the mother early in pregnancy treats the infant, preventing congenital syphilis. However, the infant needs further evaluation if the mother's treatment is within 30 days prior to delivery.

Human immunodeficiency virus infection

The effect of human immunodeficiency virus (HIV) on pregnancy outcome has produced conflicting results. HIV infection may increase the risk of stillbirth, but many in the medical profession feel that it has no effect on pregnancy outcome [23].

HIV can be transmitted to the infant *in utero*, at delivery, and by breastfeeding. The majority of cases of transmission are during delivery. The level of transmission depends mainly on the maternal HIV viral load. Higher viral loads are associated with an increased risk of transmission. Prior to the routine use of antiretroviral therapy the vertical transmission rate was about 13% in Europe in non-breastfeeding women. Breastfeeding adds a further 15% (approximately) to the transmission rate. With combination antiretroviral therapy and/or elective CS, the transmission rates can be reduced to less than 2% [24,25].

In resource rich countries, pediatric HIV infection is now a potentially preventable disease because of improved detection of the maternal infection, appropriate prenatal treatment of infected mothers, and advice not to breastfeed. In 1994, zidovudine administered to the mother in pregnancy, during delivery, and to the infant postnatally was shown to reduce vertical transmission by 68%. As the standard of care for antiretroviral therapy is now a minimum of three drugs, many pregnant women are given combination antiretroviral therapy. These treatments should be initiated by 28 weeks' gestation to obtain maximum benefit [26]. In women who have not received antenatal antiretroviral therapy, intrapartum treatment, with postpartum treatment of the infant, can still significantly lower transmission [26]. The use of neonatal postexposure prophylaxis, in the absence of maternal treatment, has not been studied in a clinical trial. Observational data suggest that zidovudine prophylaxis significantly reduces transmission if it is initiated within 48 hours of birth. There have been no trials of combination antiretroviral therapy in neonates but, in the setting of postexposure prophylaxis, three drugs are usually given for 4–6 weeks.

Studies have shown that elective CS reduces transmission by 50%–87% in women receiving no antiretroviral therapy. Combination antiretroviral therapy can reduce the maternal viral load below the level of detection. As vertical transmission seems to be extremely low with such low viral loads, it is debatable whether there is any additional benefit from CS in women taking combination antiretroviral therapy. The role of CS may be more appropriate for women receiving no antiretroviral therapy or those who are unable to achieve an undetectable viral load. After birth, the mother should not breastfeed if formula feeding can safely be given. However, in developing countries where clean water is not available, breastfeeding should continue.

The benefit of preventing vertical transmission is at the expense of exposing numerous infants to potentially toxic drugs. The long-term risks of *in utero* exposure are unknown. Short-term data on zidovudine safety are encouraging [27]. Congenital abnormalities, preterm deliveries, and low birth weights have been shown to be the same in zidovudine groups and placebo groups. A limited number of infants have now had a 6-year follow-up with no problems being reported. Given the fatal nature of HIV infection, the balance of risks is clearly in favor of antiretroviral therapy.

A woman cannot make informed choices about transmission prevention unless she knows her HIV status. Widespread antenatal HIV testing has now been introduced in many countries, including the UK. This has already resulted in a decrease in vertically transmitted HIV infection. It is anticipated that antenatal HIV testing should lead to an 80% reduction in the number of cases of vertical transmission by December 2002 [28].

Group B streptococcus

The genital and gastrointestinal tracts of approximately 20% of women are colonized by group B streptococcus (GBS). These women are predominantly asymptomatic. However, pregnant women colonized by GBS have an increased risk of preterm birth, particularly at less than 28 weeks' gestation [29]. In one study, treatment with erythromycin during pregnancy in women with GBS colonization failed to reduce preterm birth. However, this study did not reduce GBS carriage which may explain the negative findings [30].

GBS infections are a major source of morbidity for preterm and full-term infants. Neonatal infection is acquired by aspiration of infected amniotic fluid or during passage through the birth canal. In industrialized countries, GBS is the main cause of sepsis in the first week of life. In the US, Canada, and Australia, intrapartum penicillins are recommended in women with fever, prolonged rupture of membranes or imminent preterm delivery, and also in those women found to have GBS on screening at 35–37 weeks' gestation. Such intervention has reduced the incidence of GBS infections in neonates by 65% [31].

References

1.   Metters JS, editor. *Chlamydia trachomatis*. Summary and conclusions of the CMO's Expert Advisory Group. London: Department of Health, 1998.

2.   Templeton A, editor. *The prevention of pelvic infection*. London: RCOG Press, 1996.

3.   Andrews WW, Goldenberg RL, Mercer B et al. The Preterm Prediction Study: association of second-trimester genitourinary chlamydia infection with subsequent spontaneous preterm birth. *Am J Obstet Gynecol* 2000;183:662–8.

4.   Hammerschlag MR. Chlamydial infections. *J Pediatr* 1989;114:727–34.

5.   Bell TA, Stamm WE, Wang SP et al. Chronic *Chlamydia trachomatis* infections in infants. *JAMA* 1992;247:400–2.

6.   Burkman RT, Tonascia JA, Atienza MF et al. Untreated endocervical gonorrhoea and endometritis following elective abortion. *Am J Obstet Gynecol* 1976;126:648–51.

7.   Elliott B, Brunham RC, Laga M et al. Maternal gonococcal infection as a preventable risk factor for low birth weight. *J Infect Dis* 1990;161:531–6.

8.   Rawstron SA, Bromberg K, Hammerschlag MR. STD in children: syphilis and gonorrhoea. *Genitourin Med* 1993;69:66–75.

9.   Watts DH, Koutsky LA, Holmes KK et al. Low risk of perinatal transmission of human papillomavirus: results from a prospective cohort study. *Am J Obstet Gynecol* 1998;178:365–73.

10. Prober CG, Sullender WM, Yasukawa LL et al. Low risk of herpes simplex virus infections in neonates exposed to the virus at the time of vaginal delivery to mothers with recurrent genital herpes simplex infection. *N Engl J Med* 1987;316:240–4.

11. Nahmias AJ, Josey WE, Naib ZN et al. Perinatal risk associated with maternal genital herpes simplex infection. *Am J Obstet Gynecol* 1971;110:825–37.

12. Arvin AM, Hensleigh PA, Prober CG et al. Failure of antepartum maternal cultures to predict the infant's risk of exposure to herpes simplex virus at delivery. *New Engl J Med* 1986;315:796–800.

13. Scott LL, Sanchez PJ, Jackson GL et al. Acyclovir suppression to prevent Caesarean delivery after first episode genital herpes. *Obstet Gynecol* 1996;87:69–73.

14. Smith JR, Cowan FM, Munday P. The management of herpes simplex virus infection in pregnancy. *Br J Obstet Gynaecol* 1998;105:255–60.

15. Whitley R, Arvin A, Prober C et al. A controlled trial comparing vidarabine with acyclovir in neonatal herpes simplex virus infections. Infectious Diseases Collaborative Antiviral Study Group. *N Engl J Med* 1991;324:444–9.

16. Hay PE, Lamont RF, Taylor-Robinson D et al. Abnormal bacterial colonisation of the genital tract and subsequent preterm delivery and late miscarriage. *BMJ* 1994;308:295–8.

17. Koumans EH, Kendrick JS. Preventing adverse sequelae of bacterial vaginosis: public health program and research agenda. CDC Bacterial Vaginosis Working Group. *Sex Transm Dis* 2001;28:292–7.

18. Ralph SG, Rutherford AJ, Wilson JD. Influence of bacterial vaginosis on conception and miscarriage in the first trimester: cohort study. *BMJ* 1999;319:220–3.

19. Hauth JC, Goldenberg RL, Andrews WW et al. Reduced incidence of preterm delivery with metronidazole and erythromycin in women with bacterial vaginosis. *N Engl J Med* 1995;333:1732–6.

20. Carey JC, Klebanoff MA, Hauth JC et al. Metronidazole to prevent preterm delivery in pregnant women with asymptomatic bacterial vaginosis. *N Engl J Med* 2000;342:534–40.

21. Cotch MF, Pastorek JG, Nugent RP et al. *Trichomonas vaginalis* associated with low birth weight and preterm delivery. *Sex Transm Dis* 1997;24:353–60.

22. Ingraham NR. The value of penicillin alone in the prevention and treatment of syphilis. *Acta Derm Venereol* 1951;31(Suppl. 24):60–88.

23. Brocklehurst P, French R. The association between maternal HIV infection and perinatal outcome: a systematic review of the literature and meta-analysis. *Br J Obstet Gynaecol* 1998;105:836–48.

24. European Mode of Delivery Collaboration. Elective caesarean section versus vaginal delivery in prevention of vertical HIV-1 transmission: a randomised clinical trial. *Lancet* 1999;353:1035–9.

25. International Perinatal HIV Group. The mode of delivery and the risk of vertical transmission of human immunodeficiency virus type 1: a meta-analysis of 15 prospective cohort studies. *N Engl J Med* 1999;340:977–87.

26. Peckham C, Newell ML. Preventing vertical transmission of HIV infection. *N Engl J Med* 2000;343:1036–7.

27. Mofenson LM, McIntyre JA. Advances and research directions in the prevention of mother-to-child HIV-1 transmission. *Lancet* 2000;355:2237–44.

28. Unlinked Anonymous Surveys Steering Group. Prevalence of HIV and hepatitis Infections in the United Kingdom, 1999. London; Department of Health, Public Health Laboratory Service, Institute of Child Health (London), Scottish Centre for Infection and Environmental Health, 2000.

29. Regan JA, Klebanoff MA, Nugent RP et al. Colonization with group B streptococci in pregnancy and adverse outcome. VIP Study Group. *Am J Obstet Gynecol* 1996;174:1354–60.

30. Klebanoff MA, Regan JA, Rao AV et al. Outcome of the Vaginal Infections and Prematurity Study: results of a clinical trial of erythromycin among pregnant women colonized with group B streptococci. *Am J Obstet Gynecol* 1995;172:1540–5.

31. Schrag SJ, Zywicki S, Farley MM et al. Group B streptococcal disease in the era of intrapartum antibiotic prophylaxis. *N Eng J Med* 2000;342:15–20.

chapter 7

Non-hormonal contraception
Marian Everett

During the act of sexual intercourse, potential problems such as pregnancy seem remote and may not happen at all. The use of a contraceptive method requires forward planning and this is a fairly negative process. The method chosen is usually the least unpleasant of a series of poor options. Individuals seek advice from many sources about contraception, including health professionals. Between 1999 and 2000, 1.2 million women and 84 000 men visited family planning clinics in England (see Figure 7.1). The primary method of birth control used varies with age (see Figure 7.2).

The ideal contraceptive method does not exist, but if it did it would have the following characteristics:

- 100% effective
- independent of user compliance
- not related to intercourse
- 100% reversible
- free of charge or inexpensive
- acceptable to all cultures and religions
- safe
- free from side effects
- free from medical intervention
- easily available
- offering protection against sexually transmitted infections (STIs)
- easy to use

Effectiveness of contraception

The effectiveness of contraception is represented statistically by the Pearl index. The Pearl index shows the number of pregnancies per 100 woman years of use, i.e. the number of women that would become pregnant if 100 women used a given

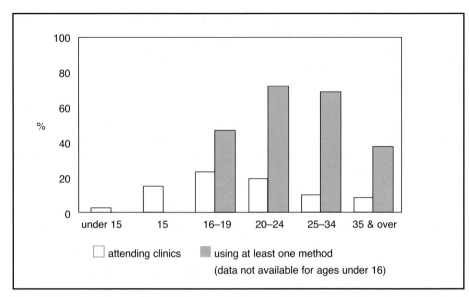

Figure 7.1 Percentage of women using at least one non-surgical method of contraception and percentage attending family planning clinics by age, 1999–2000. Source: Statistical Bulletin [4].

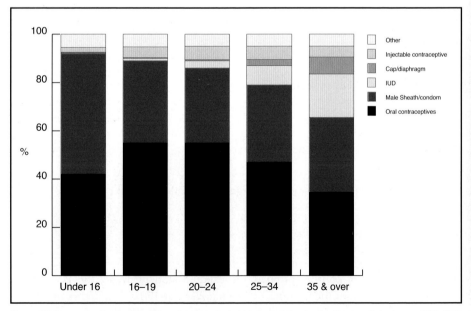

Figure 7.2 Percentage distribution of the primary method of birth control at family planning clinics by age, 1999–2000. Source: Statistical Bulletin [4]. IUD: intrauterine device.

method of family planning for 1 year. The Pearl index can be calculated using the following formula:

$$\text{Pearl index} = \frac{\text{Total number of accidental pregnancies x 1200}}{\text{Total number of months of exposure}}$$

Calculating the Pearl index involves the pooling of data, and every known conception must be included. It does not allow for women who discontinue their contraception or those who use different methods for variable durations in different studies. Fertility decreases with increasing age and all methods of contraception are more effective as women get older.

Non-hormonal contraceptive options

FERTILITY AWARENESS AND NATURAL FAMILY PLANNING

These methods rely on avoiding intercourse during the fertile phase of the cycle. A combination of factors are used such as assessing the cervical mucus, charting the longest and shortest cycles over a 6-month period and then calculating the fertile phase, and measuring the basal body temperature. A recent paper has shown that the timing of the fertile period is very variable [1]. Even in a woman with a regular cycle there is a small possibility that she will be fertile on the day that her next period is expected and 2% of women can be in the fertile phase by day 4 of the cycle.

THE PERSONA PERSONAL CONTRACEPTIVE SYSTEM

This computerized monitor measures urine levels of luteinizing hormone and estrone-3-glucuronide (see Figure 7.3). A red light on the monitor indicates the fertile time and a green light gives the go ahead for sex. Women using this method must have a cycle length between 23 and 35 days. It is unsuitable for use at the extremes of fertility, i.e. in adolescents and perimenopausal women; women who are breastfeeding; or for two cycles after childbirth, miscarriage, or abortion. It is also contraindicated for at least two cycles after any hormonal contraceptive method, including emergency contraception. The failure rate has been reported to be 6%, i.e. there is a 1 in 17 chance of pregnancy within a year of use (manufacturer's data).

COITUS INTERRUPTUS

Withdrawal, the oldest method of birth control, is still widely used and has many advantages:

- it is free from side effects and medical intervention
- it cannot be left at home!
- it is free of charge

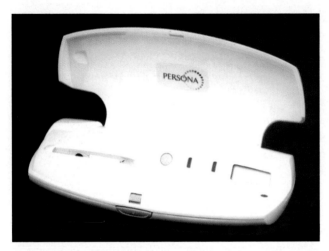

Figure 7.3 The PERSONA personal contraceptive system.

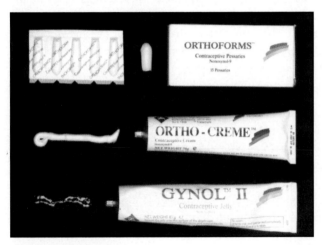

Figure 7.4 Spermicides.

However, the pre-ejaculate may contain sperm, making it a relatively ineffective method. In 1947, the Royal Commission on Population in England found that 43% of newly married couples were using withdrawal as their sole method of contraception and the pregnancy rate was found to be 8 per 100 woman years of exposure [2]. While this option should not be promoted, it is better than nothing. If *coitus interruptus* is the only acceptable option then its effectiveness can be increased by using a spermicide (see Figure 7.4).

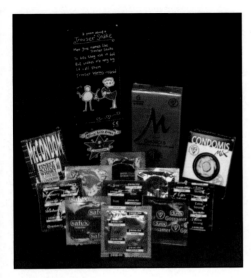

Figure 7.5 Condoms.

CONDOMS

Approximately 40 million couples worldwide rely on condoms as their only method of contraception (see Figure 7.5). Efficacy varies depending on the age (fertility) of the female partner, the frequency of intercourse, and the experience of users. Reported failure rates range from 4 to 23 pregnancies per 100 woman years. Trussell demonstrated a range of 3–12% [3].

Condoms can be obtained easily. They are inexpensive, can be widely obtained from a variety of outlets, or are free from family planning clinics. They have no side effects and protect against STIs. However, they do have some disadvantages. Most importantly, their use requires the interruption of intercourse and a high degree of motivation and care. There is also a possibility that they may slip off or burst.

FEMALE BARRIER METHODS

These include diaphragms, cervical caps, and female condoms (see Figure 7.6). Diaphragms and caps should be fitted by trained personnel and are used in conjunction with spermicides. Diaphragms fit over the entire vaginal vault and cervical caps fit on the cervix only. They are somewhat messy to use and should be left in position for at least 6 hours after intercourse. Female condoms are available over the counter and provide a very effective barrier against STIs if used correctly. There is potential for the penis to go between the device and the vaginal wall thereby rendering it ineffective.

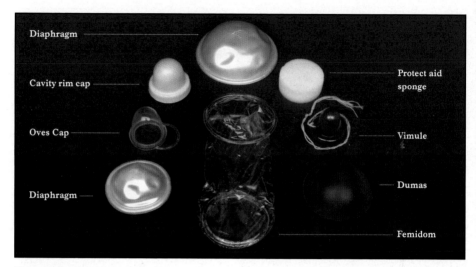

Figure 7.6 Female barrier methods of contraception.

THE INTRAUTERINE DEVICE

An intrauterine device (IUD) was used by 7% of female patients at family planning clinics in England between 1999 and 2000 [3,4]. An IUD is a solid object, usually T-shaped, which is inserted into the uterus via the vagina by a healthcare professional who has been trained in intrauterine techniques. A thread is attached to the base of the device to allow for easy removal. Inert (plastic) devices are no longer used in the UK and all current devices are copper bearing (see Figure 7.7). The progestogen-releasing intrauterine system (Mirena) is discussed in the section on hormonal contraceptive options. IUD types that are commonly used in the UK and their effectiveness are provided in Table 7.1.

Device	Licensed lifespan (years)	Pearl index
Multiload 250	3	1–2
Multiload 335	5	0.5
Nova-T	5	1–3
Nova-T 380	5	0.5
Flexi-T	3	1–3
GyneFIX	5	0.5
T-safe 380A	8	0.5

Table 7.1 Intrauterine device types commonly used in the UK.

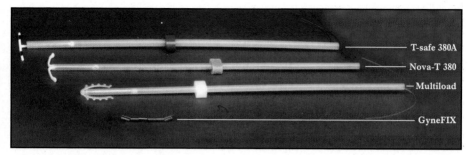

Figure 7.7 The intrauterine device.

Mode of action

Copper coils are associated with a whole range of cellular and biochemical changes (see Table 7.2). The major mode of action is to impede the transport of spermatozoa during the prefertilization phase. Copper is toxic to sperm, ova, and the developing blastocyst, and also increases prostaglandin levels. The physical presence of the device induces a foreign body reaction resulting in biochemical changes in the endometrium that lead to the disruption of enzyme systems and hormone receptors. Because of this foreign body reaction, the white blood cell concentration in the endometrium and the uterine and tubal fluids is increased. Phagocytosis of sperm has been observed. Although the main effect of copper IUDs is to block fertilization, an implantation blocking effect has also been observed as shown by the efficacy of a postcoital IUD as a contraception option when inserted up to 5 days after ovulation (see Chapter 8).

Copper is toxic to sperm, ova, and the blastocyst
Increased foreign body reaction
Leukocytosis with phagocytosis of sperm
Raised prostaglandin levels

Table 7.2 Mode of action of copper bearing intrauterine devices.

Efficacy

The overall failure rate is 0.2 to 3 per 100 woman years (see Table 7.1). In women over 35 years the failure rate is 0.1 to 0.5 per 100 woman years.

Advantages and disadvantages

Prior to the fitting of an IUD, a full explanation of the risks and benefits must be given to each woman and informed consent obtained. The IUD is an excellent method of contraception. Modern devices are highly effective at protecting against pregnancy and can be fitted up to 5 days after the expected date of ovulation in any woman. They can also be fitted immediately after surgical termination or evacuation of the uterus. Postnatally, they can be fitted at 4 weeks or 6–8 weeks following a Cesarean section and they have no effect on lactation. They do not rely on user compliance and are independent of intercourse. They have high continuance rates and are easily reversible. Any copper device fitted in women over the age of 40 years can remain *in situ* until 1 year after the menopause without needing to be changed [5].

There is a small failure rate (see Table 7.1), and if a pregnancy should occur there is an increased risk of miscarriage. During the fitting procedure the incidence of uterine perforation is 1 in 1000 [6]. Pelvic inflammatory disease is caused primarily by a sexually acquired infection and the risk of developing the condition is greatest during the first 20 days after fitting an IUD [5]. The risks can be minimized by screening all women for chlamydia and administering prophylactic antibiotics (azithromycin [1 g] or doxycycline [100 mg] twice daily for 7 days) at the time of fitting. The partners of chlamydia-positive women should be contacted and treated. Advantages and disadvantages of using an IUD as a contraceptive method are summarized in Table 7.3.

Advantages	Disadvantages
• Effective	• Risk of miscarriage if failure occurs
• Safe	• Risk of perforation during fitting
• Does not rely on user compliance	• Risk of expulsion
• Independent of intercourse	• Longer heavier periods
• Reversible	• Dysmenorrhea
• Cheap	• No protection against sexually
• Can be used during lactation	transmitting infections

Table 7.3 Advantages and disadvantages of intrauterine devices.

Ectopic pregnancy and IUDs
Copper IUDs do not increase the overall risk of ectopic pregnancy in the population but they do increase the relative risk of ectopic pregnancy. The background risk of ectopic pregnancy is 1 in 100, i.e. if 1000 women become pregnant, 10 will have an ectopic pregnancy (giving a ratio of 1:100). If 1000 women are using an IUD with a failure rate of 1 in 100, 10 women will become pregnant. Of these 10 pregnancies, one will be ectopic (giving a ratio of 1:10) [7]. Women who experience an ectopic pregnancy usually have pre-existing tubal damage from pelvic infection.

Contraindications

In 1994, the World Health Organization (WHO) developed a classification system for contraindications to contraceptive use (see Table 7.4) [8]. For every individual woman the health care provider must make an assessment of the risks and benefits of the contraceptive method to be used and must counsel the client accordingly.

WHO grade 1 condition	A condition for which there is no restriction on use
WHO grade 2 condition	A condition where the advantages generally outweigh the risks
WHO grade 3 condition	A condition where the risks generally outweigh the advantages
WHO grade 4 condition	A condition which represents an unacceptable health risk

Table 7.4 The WHO classification system for medical eligibility criteria for contraceptive use [8].

Contraindications for IUD use

WHO grade 4 conditions
- suspicion of pregnancy
- undiagnosed vaginal bleeding
- current pelvic infection
- post-septic abortion
- immunosupression
- trophoblastic disease
- a markedly distorted uterine cavity
- allergy to any of the constituents of the IUD
- Wilson's disease
- past history of bacterial endocarditis in a woman with an anatomical heart lesion
- presence of a prosthetic heart valve

WHO grade 3 conditions
- immediately after delivery
- past history of ectopic pregnancy
- past history of tubal surgery
- menorrhagia
- severe primary dysmenorrhea

However, most women can be fitted with an IUD. Nulliparity or a young age are not contraindications. All women need careful counseling about the risks and benefits of intrauterine contraception. The fitting procedure must be discussed prior to obtaining informed consent.

References

1.   Wilcox AJ, Dunson D, Baird DD et al. The timing of the 'fertile window' in the menstrual cycle: day specific estimates from a prospective study. *BMJ* 2000;321:1259–62.

2.   Notestein FW. The report of the Royal Commission on Population: a review. In: Population Studies, Volume 3, 1949/1950:232–40.

3.   Trussell J. Contraceptive failure rates 1994. In: Hatcher RA, Trussell J, Stewart F, editors. *Contraceptive technology*. 17th revised edition. New York: Irvington Publishers, 1998:637–87.

4.   NHS Contraceptive Services, England: 1999–2000. Statistical Bulletin. Available at: URL: http://www.doh.gov.uk/pdfs/sb0027.pdf.

5.   Newton J, Tacchi D. Long-term use of copper intrauterine devices. A statement from the Medical Advisory Committee of the Family Planning Association and the National Association of Family Planning Doctors. *Lancet* 1990;335:1322-3.

6.   Glasier A, Gebbie A. Handbook of Family Planning and Reproductive Healthcare. 4th edition. Churchill Livingstone, 2000:112.

7.   Guillebaud J. Contraception: Your Questions Answered. 3rd ed. Edinburgh: Churchill Livingstone, 1999:353.

8.   World Health Organization. Improved access to quality care in family planning: medical eligibility criteria for contraceptive use. WHO/FRH/FPP/96.9.

chapter 8

Hormonal contraception

Marian Everett

Hormonal contraception includes the combined oral contraceptive (COC) pill, the progestogen-only pill (POP), implants, injections, and the hormone-releasing intrauterine system (IUS).

Oral contraceptives

According to the general household survey in 1995, oral contraception is used by 25% of the 13 million women between the ages of 16–49 in the UK [1]. In England in 1999, 0.4 million women were prescribed the oral contraceptive pill by family planning clinics and 2.6 million prescriptions were written by general practitioners (10% were for the POP) [2].

THE COMBINED ORAL CONTRACEPTIVE PILL
Mode of action

Ovulation of maturing follicles in the ovary is induced by a large burst of luteinizing hormone (LH) secretion, known as the LH surge. The COC pill prevents ovulation by halting follicular maturation and abolishing the estrogen-mediated positive feedback mechanism that triggers the LH surge. It also induces a thickening of the cervical mucus, making it impenetrable to sperm, and alters the endometrium, making it unreceptive to blastocyst implantation.

Types of COC pills

All COC pills contain the estrogen, ethinyl estradiol, and a progestogen. One active pill is taken every 24 hours for 21 days out of 28. Everyday brands also contain seven placebo tablets. COC pills may be of a fixed dose (a constant dose of estrogen and progestogen in each tablet), biphasic (one change in dose over the course of the cycle), or triphasic (two changes in dose). The dose of ethinyl estradiol ranges from 20–50 μg, with most pills containing 30 or 35 μg.

The first progestogen to be synthesized was norethisterone in 1950, but there is now a wide range of different progestogens available. Norethisterone and levonorgestrel have androgenic side effects – e.g. acne and hair growth – and also reduce the levels of

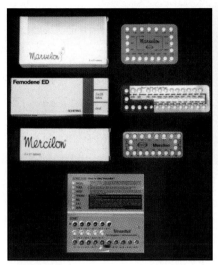

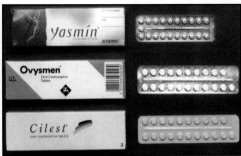

Figure 8.1 Different combined oral contraceptive pills.

high-density lipoproteins, potentially resulting in an increased susceptibility to arterial disease with long-term use. The newer progestogens – desogestrel, norgestimate, and gestodene – have very weak androgenic or even antiandrogenic activity (reducing acne and facial hair growth). Drospirenone, another new progestogen, has recently been developed with potent progestogenic, antimineralocorticoid, and antiandrogenic properties. Drospirenone is a derivative of spironolactone. Its antimineralocorticoid activity induces a negative sodium balance with small reductions in blood pressure and weight. It reverses the estrogen induced fluid retention caused by sodium retention and increased plasma volume. Studies demonstrate that women have either a stable body weight or a slight decrease in weight [3]. This may be an important factor in improving compliance in some women. Drospirenone has been combined with 30 μg of ethinyl estradiol in a new COC pill, Yasmin, which was launched in the UK in 2002. Examples of different types of COC pills are provided in Figure 8.1 and their properties are provided in Table 8.1.

Progestogen	Androgenic	Antiandrogenic	Antimineralocorticoid
Norethisterone	Yes	No	No
Levonorgestrel	Yes	No	No
Desogestrel	No	Yes	No
Norgestimate	Weak	No	No
Gestodene	Weak	No	No
Drospirenone	No	Yes	Yes

Table 8.1 Types and properties of progestogens available in combined oral contraceptives.

Starting the COC

The COC pill can be started on days 1–5 of the menstrual cycle. However, if it is started after day 2, then additional barrier contraception should be used for 7 days. The COC pill can be started immediately following a miscarriage or termination of pregnancy. Postpartum, the COC pill can be started on day 21 by non-breast-feeding women. It is unsuitable for use by lactating women as it can suppress milk production.

Efficacy

The COC pill has a failure rate of 0.1% with perfect use, increasing to 5% with typical use [4]. Modern pills containing 30–35 μg of ethinyl estradiol are only just sufficient to prevent conception in some women. Because of this reduced margin for error, any minor deviations of compliance can lead to failure [5].

Reduced efficacy

The efficacy of COCs is reduced by vomiting within 2 hours of taking the tablet, or by severe diarrhea. The use of condoms should be advised during gastrointestinal upset and for 7 days following recovery.

Broadspectrum antibiotics including penicillins, ampicillin, cephalosporins, and tetracyclines, alter bowel flora and may affect the enterohepatic recirculation of ethinyl estradiol. Condoms should be used whilst taking these medications and for 7 days following recovery. Long-term antibiotics, e.g. tetracycline for acne, require the concomitant use of a condom for the first few weeks of treatment. However, there are other antibiotics such as trimethoprim and metronidazole that do not affect the efficacy of COCs because they do not alter bowel flora.

Enzyme-inducing drugs can have very long-acting effects on the COCs. Examples of these drugs include rifampicin, griseofulvin, phenobarbitone, phenytoin, and carbamazepine. Women who are taking these drugs long term are advised to use alternative methods of contraception, e.g. IUDs, or Depo-Provera at 8-week intervals instead of twelve.

For short courses of enzyme-inducing drugs, the use of condoms should be advised for one month following completion of therapy.

Missed pills

The COC pill should be taken regularly every 24 hours for 21 days out of 28. Pills that are taken more than 12 hours late are counted as missed pills. During the pill-free interval, ovarian follicular activity starts to resume so that ovulation may occur if pills are missed at the beginning or end of a packet. Two or more missed pills in the first week of pill taking, or four or more missed pills in the second week, may result in a breakthrough ovulation. If pills are missed in the third week, then the next packet should be started immediately without a pill-free interval.

Advantages and disadvantages of the COC pill are provided in Table 8.2.

Advantages	Disadvantages
• Effective	• Minor side effects such as acne, breast tenderness, leg cramps, and headaches
• Convenient	
• Reversible	• Nausea and weight gain
• Reduced menstrual flow [6]	• A small increased risk of breast cancer [8]
• Reduced anemia [6]	
• Protection against pelvic inflammatory disease (PID) [7]	• Venous thromboembolus [9]
	• Arterial disease
• Reduced risk of benign breast disease [6]	• Not suitable for use during lactation
• Reduced risk of ovarian and endometrial carcinoma	

Table 8.2 Advantages and disadvantages of the combined oral contraceptive pill.

Contraindications
World Health Organization (WHO) grade 4 conditions
Conditions that represent an unacceptable health risk.

Circulatory disease
- past proven venous or arterial thrombosis
- ischemic heart disease
- angina
- all cardiomyopathies
- severe risk factors for venous or arterial disease
- known atherogenic lipid disorders
- congenital or acquired thrombophilia
- scleroderma and systemic lupus erythematosus
- migraine with focal aura
- structural or uncorrected valvular heart disease

Liver disease
- active liver disease
- history of cholestatic jaundice of pregnancy
- Dubin–Johnson and Roter syndromes
- acute porphyrias
- untreated gallstones
- liver tumors

Other
- possible pregnancy
- undiagnosed vaginal bleeding
- estrogen-dependent tumor
- benign intracranial hypertension
- trophoblastic disease with raised human chorionic gonadotropin (hCG) levels
- otosclerosis

WHO grade 3 conditions
Conditions where the disadvantages of COC use generally outweigh the advantages.
- risk factors for circulatory disease, e.g. essential hypertension
- long-term immobilization, e.g. wheelchair users
- severe depression
- splenectomy (platelets must be monitored)
- diabetes mellitus
- inflammatory bowel disease

Management of common problems
Minor side effects are commonly described by women taking the COC pill. These include breakthrough bleeding (BTB), acne, headaches, weight gain, and low libido.

Breakthrough bleeding
BTB commonly occurs within the first 2–3 months of pill taking. New pill users should be counseled to expect this, though it does usually settle. Persistent BTB after 3 months of taking the COC pill, or the onset of BTB after several months of regular withdrawal, needs to be investigated.

Poor compliance – pills taken late or missed completely – often leads to BTB. Another common cause is drug interactions. Prescription medicines that are enzyme-inducers, e.g. carbamazepine, rifampicin, and some over-the-counter products such as St. John's wort, can affect the metabolism of the COC causing BTB and reduced protection against pregnancy. Diarrhea and vomiting can impair the absorption of the COC and lead to BTB. Cervical problems – in particular undiagnosed chlamydial infection – can lead to spotting, BTB, and postcoital bleeding. A sexual history should be taken, and a pelvic examination and inspection performed. Endocervical swabs should also be taken to exclude chlamydia and gonorrhea. A cervical smear test is only necessary if one is due. A smear is not a diagnostic test for women with symptoms, but a screening tool for asymptomatic women. If the cervix looks suspicious in any way, then a referral for colposcopy should be made.

When all of these causes of BTB have been excluded, it may be useful to change the type of COC. Changing from a monophasic pill to a triphasic pill containing the same progestogen, e.g. Microgynon to Logynon, may result in better cycle control. Increasing the estrogen content may also be beneficial, e.g. changing to Ovran 50, or prescribing two Microgynon 30 tablets/day, but this is an unlicensed use and must be done on a 'named patient' basis only.

Acne
Women with pre-existing acne should be given a less androgenic pill (see Table 8.1). Dianette – a combination of 35 μg ethinyl estradiol and 2 mg cyproterone acetate – is licensed for the treatment of severe acne, and can be very effective after several months of use. It also provides contraception. Preliminary studies have demonstrated that Yasmin, the newest COC available, is also very effective in the treatment of acne [10].

Headaches and migraine
Pre-existing migraine with focal aura, or first-time occurrence of migraine whilst taking the COC, is a WHO grade 4 condition and a contraindication for the COC.

Headaches are a common side effect of the COC, and often occur during the pill-free interval due to sudden decreases in circulating hormone levels. It is possible to manage these headaches by tricycling the pill, i.e. running three packets together. This should reduce the number of cycles and, therefore, the number of headaches. Headaches that occur on pill-taking days should be managed by prescribing the lowest acceptable monophasic regime, e.g. Mercilon Femodette. If headaches persist, switching to a progestogen-only method will often resolve the problem.

Weight gain and bloating
Weight gain is often attributed to the use of hormonal contraception. However, many young women start taking the COC at a time when they are still growing, and a steady increase in weight during teenage years is absolutely normal. Some women complain of an increase in appetite whilst taking the COC. If dietary advice and exercise do not

help, then switching to a low-dose pill (e.g. Mercilon Femodette), or an alternative method (e.g. the POP) may be necessary.

Bloating may occur due to fluid retention; the excess fluid is shed during the pill-free week. As this tends to be linked with estrogen, a progestogen-dominant pill, e.g. Loestrin 30 or Microgynon 30, may reduce the likelihood of bloating.

Loss of libido

Some women will find an increase in libido due to the relief of premenstrual syndrome, and the confidence gained from the reliability of this method. However, other women will report loss of libido after starting the COC pill. This may be unrelated to the COC, so a full history should be taken to include details of the relationship and psychosexual aspects, as it may be necessary to refer the woman for counseling. Vaginal problems causing dyspareunia, e.g. soreness and dryness, should be eliminated first. Switching to an estrogen-dominant pill (e.g. Ovysmen or Marvelon) may help to prevent loss of libido.

THE PROGESTOGEN-ONLY PILL

The POP, or the mini pill, is taken by approximately 10% of the 3 million women using oral contraception in England [2]. It consists of a small continuous dose of progestogen taken daily. Currently there are six POPs available in the UK (see Table 8.3 and Figure 8.2). Efficacy depends upon the age and motivation of the user. Meticulous care and use of an additional barrier method, if indicated, are required to ensure that the method is effective.

Mode of action

The POP alters the cervical mucus, making it impenetrable to sperm. Diminished follicular activity and low estradiol levels are evident in 16% of women; these women will not ovulate [5].

Name of pill	Progestogen	Dose (μg)
Microval	Levonorgestrel	30
Norgeston	Levonorgestrel	30
Neogest	Levonorgestrel	37.5
Cerazette	Desogestral	75
Micronor	Norethisterone	350
Noriday	Norethisterone	350
Femulen	Ethynodiol diacetate	500

Table 8.3 The progestogen type and dosage used in progestogen-only pills.

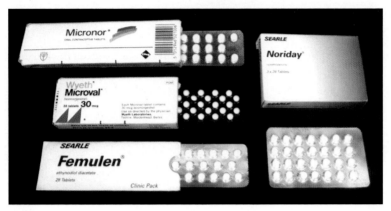

Figure 8.2 Different progestogen-only pills.

Starting the POP

The POP can be started on days 1–5 of the menstrual cycle. However, if it is started after day 2, then additional barrier contraception should be used for the next 7 days. If changing from the COC pill to the POP, then the first POP should be taken on the day following the last COC pill. The POP may be started immediately following a miscarriage or termination of pregnancy. Postpartum, it can be started between days 21–28 and can be used during lactation.

Efficacy

Efficacy depends upon the motivation and age of the user. The Pearl index varies from 0.3 to 4 per 100 woman years. The failure rate is influenced by age and has been reported to be 3.1 per 100 in the 25–29 age group [4] and 0.3 per 100 in those over 40 years old [4]. In lactating women the POP is almost 100% effective.

Reduced efficacy

The efficacy of the POP is reduced by vomiting within 2 hours of taking the tablet, or by severe diarrhea, indicating the need for additional barrier contraception for 7 days following recovery.

Unlike the COC pill, the efficacy of the POP is not affected by broadspectrum antibiotics. However, it is still not recommended for women who are taking long-term drugs that activate liver enzymes, e.g. rifampicin, phenobarbitone, or carbamazepine.

To remain effective, the POP must be taken regularly every 24 hours. A pill taken more than 3 hours late requires the use of additional barrier contraception for the next 7 days. Advantages and disadvantages of the POP are provided in Table 8.4.

Advantages	Disadvantages
• Effective—especially in older and breastfeeding women • Safe—there is no evidence of an increased risk of coronary heart disease or malignant disease • Can be used by women in whom estrogen is contraindicated • Rapid return of fertility after discontinuation • Some protection against pelvic infection due to cervical mucus effects	• Efficacy depends on user compliance —the pills must be taken regularly and additional use of a barrier method is required for 7 days if any pill is taken more than 3 hours late • Alteration of the menstrual pattern— anything from amenorrhea to unpredictable chaotic bleeding can occur • Functional ovarian cysts are common and occur in about half of all POP users • Reduced risk of ectopic pregnancy in POP users compared with sexually active non-pregnant controls, but if a breakthrough pregnancy should occur then the chance of it being ectopic is increased

Table 8.4 Advantages and disadvantages of the progestogen-only pill.

Contraindications

WHO grade 4 conditions

- current ischemic heart disease, angina, or thrombotic stroke
- severe hereditary lipid disorders
- cholestatic jaundice of pregnancy
- liver tumors
- current liver disease
- trophoblastic disease with raised hCG levels
- acute porphyrias
- pregnancy
- undiagnosed vaginal bleeding

WHO grade 3 conditions
- previous ectopic pregnancy
- history of functional ovarian cysts
- severe risk factors for arterial disease
- past subarachnoid hemorrhage
- hormone-dependent cancer (breast cancer)

Injectable hormonal contraception

DEPO-PROVERA

Depo-Provera is a long-acting hormonal form of birth control where the active agent is a synthetic progestogen (depot-medroxyprogesterone acetate) (see Figure 8.3). A 150 mg deep intramuscular injection is administered every 11–12 weeks. The first injection must be given within the first 5 days after the beginning of a period (unless the client is already using the pill or has an intrauterine device [IUD]) or within the first 5 days after an abortion or miscarriage. After childbirth it may be given in the first week after delivery but can cause problems with menorrhagia and it is usually delayed until 4–5 weeks post-delivery. The level of hormone gradually declines over the 12-week period and a repeat injection is required. This method was used by 6% of attendees at English family planning clinics between 1999 and 2000 [4].

Mode of action

Depo-Provera prevents ovulation and induces changes to the endometrium that make implantation less likely. The cervical mucus becomes thicker making it more difficult for sperm to enter the uterus.

Contraindications

WHO grade 4 conditions
- past arterial disease
- current active liver disease
- acute porphyria
- liver tumor
- past history of cholestatic jaundice of pregnancy
- pregnancy
- undiagnosed vaginal bleeding
- trophoblastic disease with raised hCG levels
- hormone-dependent malignancies

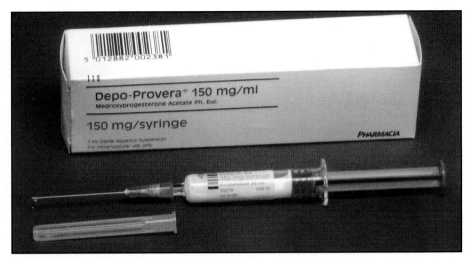

Figure 8.3 Depo-Provera.

WHO grade 3 conditions
- unacceptability of unpredictable bleeding pattern
- planning a pregnancy in the near future
- past history of severe depression

Efficacy
The Pearl index is estimated to be 0.1 per 100 woman years. Advantages and disadvantages of Depo-Provera are provided in Table 8.5.

Depo-Provera and bone density
Depo-Provera suppresses ovulation and estradiol levels are low (<150 pmol/L) in long-term users. Low estradiol levels are associated with low bone density. As early as 1991, a paper was published showing that long-term users of Depo-Provera had lower bone densities than premenopausal controls [11]. In 1994, the same research group confirmed that the bone loss was completely reversed 2 years after discontinuation of Depo-Provera [12].

Teenage girls using Depo-Provera were shown to have a mean decrease in bone density of 3.1% over 2 years [13]. However, Gbolade et al. showed that a group of British women who used Depo-Provera had bone densities only minimally below the normal population mean with no correlation between estradiol levels and bone density [14].

Advantages	Disadvantages
• Highly effective	• Severe disturbances of menstruation
• Convenient	• It is reversible eventually but it can take time (up to 9 months) for effects to wear off
• Reversible	
• Amenorrhea (less anemia)	
• Reduced incidence of PID	• Weight gain
• Protection against endometrial carcinoma	• Side effects such as mood swings, bloating, or breast tenderness
• Fewer crises in patients with sickle cell disease	• Cannot be removed or reversed once given
• Can be used while breastfeeding	
• Can be used when estrogen is contraindicated	
• Minimal effect on lipids	
• Minimal effect on clotting factors	

Table 8.5 Advantages and disadvantages of Depo-Provera.

The available data for women aged between 20–40 years would suggest that bone density is lower in long-term users but it reverses quickly once Depo-Provera has been discontinued. Very young women, i.e. aged 16 years or younger, who still have not achieved their peak bone mass have been included in the WHO grade 2 conditions group where the advantages of use usually outweigh the risks. Nonetheless, there are concerns about bone density in this group. For older women, i.e. over 45 years old, and especially smokers, the risks may start to outweigh the benefits, and these women should be carefully counseled about the risk of osteoporosis as they approach the menopause.

Management of late attendance for Depo-Provera

According to the manufacturer's guidelines, protection from pregnancy is lost at 12 weeks and five days (89 days) after the previous injection. Many providers of contraceptive services have a reminder system to notify women who fail to attend at 11 weeks for repeat injections. The majority of women will have amenorrhea whilst using Depo-Provera, and this may continue for 6–12 months after the last injection. Thus, waiting for the onset of the next menses, in order to administer the next

Attendance	Management
Up to 89 days	Administer next Depo-Provera injection—no extra precautions necessary
89–92 days	If unprotected intercourse has taken place within 72 hours, offer emergency contraception and Depo-Provera.
	If there has been no intercourse, advise extra precautions for 7 days, and a pregnancy test at 3 weeks.
92–94 days	If unprotected intercourse has taken place between 72 hours and 5 days, offer a copper IUD and a Depo-Provera injection.
	At a follow-up appointment 2–3 weeks later, perform a pregnancy test and remove the coil.
94 days onwards	Carry out a pregnancy test. If result is negative, advise abstinence from intercourse for the next 14 days and then repeat pregnancy test. If test is negative again, administer Depo-Provera injection and advise extra precautions for 7 days.

Table 8.6 The management of late attendance for Depo-Provera [15].

injection, should be avoided, as during this time, pregnancy may ensue. The management of late attendance for Depo-Provera is summarized in Table 8.6.

NORETHISTERONE ENANTHATE

A 200 mg intramuscular injection is given every 8 weeks. It is only licensed for short-term use in the UK, i.e. two injections 2 months apart. It may be used on a long-term basis in some patients. It is less likely than Depo-Provera to produce amenorrhea and there is a reduced chance of weight gain. Some women find this form of contraception more acceptable than others but the injection is painful because it is oil based. Norethisterone enanthate works by inhibiting ovulation.

SUBDERMAL IMPLANTS

Implanon (see Figure 8.4) is now the only contraceptive implant available in the UK. It should be fitted during the first 5 days of the cycle in women who are not using contraception, but can be fitted at any time in women using effective contraception,

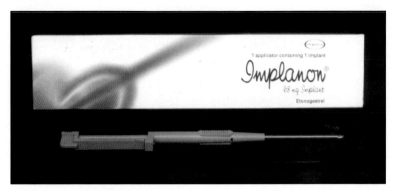

Figure 8.4. The Implanon subdermal implant.

e.g. COC pills, POPs, or coils. Implanon consists of a single flexible rod composed of ethylene vinyl acetate. The rod is impregnated with 68 μg of the progestogen, etonogestrel, and a small amount is released every day. It is inserted just under the skin on the inside of the upper arm and provides 3 years of highly effective contraception [14]. Norplant, a six rod contraceptive implant releasing levonorgestrel, was withdrawn from the UK market in 1999.

Mode of action
The principal mode of action of Implanon is to inhibit ovulation by preventing the LH surge. It also affects the cervical mucus, making it impenetrable to sperm, and induces endometrial changes, discouraging implantation.

Efficacy
The Pearl index is 0.8 per 100 woman years. Advantages and disadvantages of Implanon are provided in Table 8.7.

Contraindications
WHO grade 4 conditions
- acute porphyria
- pregnancy
- undiagnosed vaginal bleeding
- hormone-dependent tumors (breast)
- acute liver disease
- active venous thromboembolic disease

Advantages	Disadvantages
• Effective • Safe • Independent of user compliance • Independent of intercourse • Amenorrhea in 25–30% of users • Suitable for women in whom estrogen is contraindicated • Rapidly reversible	• Minor side effects such as weight gain, mood swings, and bloating • Effects on the bleeding pattern are variable—from amenorrhea to chaotic progestogen-type bleeding • Minor surgical procedure required for insertion and removal

Table 8.7 Advantages and disadvantages of subdermal implants.

WHO grade 3 conditions
- unacceptability of irregular bleeding patterns
- obesity – uncertainty about the efficiency of this method in the final year of use in obese women

The Mirena intrauterine system

The Mirena IUS is a T-shaped IUD (see Figure 8.5) that releases 20 μg of levonorgestrel per day from a polydimethyl siloxane reservoir. It is licensed for 5 years use in the UK. A much lower dose of levonorgestrel is released than with the pill and it acts directly on the endometrium. Systemic side effects such as bloating, mood swings, and acne occasionally occur in the first 2 months after insertion but these usually settle down with time. The Mirena IUS should be fitted during the first 5 days of the menstrual cycle in women who are not currently using an alternative contraception.

MODE OF ACTION
The main effect of the Mirena IUS is on the endometrium. This becomes inactive with atrophy of the glands, suppression of spiral arterioles, and capillary thrombosis. The cervical mucus also becomes impenetrable to sperm.

Efficacy
Mirena is highly effective. A recent UK study reported a Pearl index of 0.6 per 100 woman years [16]. As with all intrauterine contraception, full counseling is required prior to obtaining informed consent to have the Mirena fitted. Advantages and disadvantages of the Mirena IUS are provided in Table 8.8.

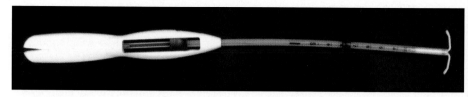

Figure 8.5 The Mirena IUS.

Advantages	Disadvantages
• Effective	• Carries the same risk of perforation, expulsion, and malpositioning as a non-progestogen-releasing IUD
• Safe	
• Reversible within one cycle	
• Reduction in menstrual blood loss [17]	• Irregular bleeding during the initial months after insertion [18]
• Independent of user compliance	
• Reduced incidence of pelvic infection	• Functional ovarian cysts

Table 8.8 Advantages and disadvantages of the Mirena IUS.

References

1. Living in Britain. Results from the 1995 General Household Survey. London: The Stationery Office, 1996.

2. NHS Contraceptive Services, England 1999–2000 Statistical Bulletin. Available at: htpp://www.doh.gov.uk/pdfs/sb0027.pdf

3. Oelkers W, Helmerhorst FM, Wuttke W et al. Effect of an oral contraceptive containing drospirenone on the renin-angiotensin-aldosterone system in healthy female volunteers. *Gynecol Endocrinol* 2000;14:204–13.

4. Trussell J. Contraceptive failure rates 1994. In: Hatcher RA, Trussell J, Stewart F, editors. *Contraceptive technology*. 17th revised edition. New York: Irvington Publishers, 1998:637–87.

5. Guillebaud J. Contraception: your questions answered. 3rd edition. Edinburgh: Churchill Livingston, 1999:102.

6. Larsson G, Milsom I, Lindstedt G et al. The influence of a low-dose combined oral contraceptive on menstrual blood loss and iron status. *Contraception* 1992;46:327–34.

7. Wolner-Hanssen P, Eschenbach DA, Paavonen J et al. Decreased risk of symptomatic chamydial pelvic inflammatory disease associated with oral contraceptive use. *JAMA* 1990;263:54–9.

8. Collaborative Group on Hormonal Factors in Breast Cancer. Breast cancer and hormone replacement therapy: collaborative reanalysis of data from 51 epidemiological studies of 52 705 women with breast cancer and 108 411 women without breast cancer. *Lancet* 1997;350:1047–59.

9. World Health Organization Collaborative Study of Cardiovascular Disease and Steroid Hormone Contraception. Effect of different progestagens in low oestrogen oral contraceptives on venous thromboembolic disease. *Lancet* 1995;346:1582–8.

10. Huber J, Foidart JM, Wuttke W et al. Efficacy and tolerability of a monophasic oral contraceptive containing ethinylestradiol and drospirenone. *Eur J Contracept Reprod Health Care* 2000;5:25–34.

11. Cundy T, Evans M, Roberts H et al. Bone density in women receiving depot medroxyprogesterone acetate for contraception. *BMJ* 1991;303:13–6.

12. Cundy T, Cornish J, Evans MC et al. Recovery of bone density in women who stop using medroxyprogesterone acetate. *BMJ* 1994;308:247–8.

13. Cromer BA, Blair JM, Mahan JD et al. A prospective comparison of bone density in adolescent girls receiving depot medroxyprogesterone (Depo-Provera), levonorgestrel (Norplant), or oral contraceptives. *J Pediatr* 1996;129:671–6.

14. Gbolade B, Ellis S, Murby B et al. Bone density in long term users of depot medroxyprogesterone acetate. *Br J Obstet Gynaecol* 1998;105:790–4.

15. Bigrigg A, Evans M. Gbolade B et al. Depo Provera. Position paper on clinical use, effectiveness and side effects. *Br J Fam Plann* 1999;25:69–76 (review).

16. Edwards JE, Moore A. Implanon. A review of clinical studies. *Brit J Fam Plann* 1999;24:3–16.

17. Bounds W, Robinson G, Kubba A et al. Clinical experience with a levonorgestrel-releasing intrauterine contraceptive device (LNG-IUD) as a contraceptive and in the treatment of menorrhagia. *Br J Fam Plann* 1993;19:193–4.

18. Cox M, Blacksell S. Clinical performance of the levonorgestrel intrauterine system in routine use by the UK Family Planning and Reproductive Health Research Network: 12-month report. *Br J Fam Plann* 2000;26:143–7.

chapter 9

Emergency contraception
Marian Everett

In England, between the years 1999 and 2000, 0.8 million prescriptions were issued for emergency contraception. The vast majority were issued by community family health clinics and general practitioners (GPs), with only 2% being issued via hospital accident and emergency (A&E) departments [1]. Emergency contraception is defined as any method that acts after coitus has taken place and prior to implantation. Implantation is assumed to occur no sooner than 5 days after ovulation. Emergency contraception has no effect after the ovum is implanted in the uterus.

Hormonal emergency contraception

The mode of action of hormonal methods depends upon the stage in the menstrual cycle when they are administered. If these methods are used early in the cycle, ovulation is delayed. If given later in the cycle, implantation is blocked by a disturbance of the endometrium and effects on estrogen and progesterone receptors. All currently licensed methods of emergency contraception are ineffective once implantation has occurred.

THE YUZPE REGIMEN
The Yuzpe regimen has been used since the 1970s. With this method, two doses of ethinyl estradiol (100 µg) plus levonorgestrel (500 µg) are taken 12 hours apart. The Yuzpe regimen has been shown to prevent 57% of expected pregnancies when initiated within 72 hours of unprotected intercourse [2]. The main side effects are nausea (51% of users) and vomiting (19% of users). PC4 was the only licensed product (in the UK) on the market but was withdrawn in 2002 (see Figure 9.1).

THE PROGESTOGEN-ONLY EMERGENCY CONTRACEPTIVE PILL
In 1998, the World Health Organization (WHO) published details of a large trial investigating the efficacy of the progestogen-only emergency contraceptive (POEC) pill [2]. It was proposed that two doses of levonorgestrel (750 µg), taken 12 hours apart, are even more effective for preventing pregnancy than the Yuzpe regimen (see Table 9.1). The POEC method has fewer side effects, causing nausea in 23% of users

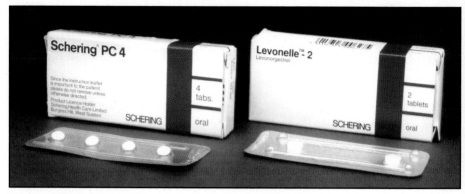

Figure 9.1 Hormonal emergency contraception—PC4 and Levonelle.

and vomiting in only 6% of users. Levonelle was launched in the UK in January, 2000 (see Figure 9.1).

Coitus to treatment interval (hours)	% of expected pregnancies prevented with the Yuzpe regimen	% of expected pregnancies prevented using POEC
≤24	77	95
25–48	36	85
48–72	31	58

Table 9.1 Efficacy of the Yuzpe regimen versus the progestogen-only emergency contraceptive pill method [2].

A more recent review of efficacy studies showed that the Yuzpe regimen would prevent up to 74% of expected pregnancies when initiated within 72 hours [3]. The discrepancy between this study and the WHO study is currently under investigation.

WHO SHOULD BE OFFERED HORMONAL EMERGENCY CONTRACEPTION?

The overall risk of pregnancy after a single act of unprotected sex on any day in the menstrual cycle is between 2–4%. The pregnancy risk is highest around the time of ovulation (20–30%). On any day of the menstrual cycle, it cannot be guaranteed that unprotected intercourse will not result in pregnancy [4]. Therefore, emergency contraception should be considered for the following groups of women:

- those who have had unprotected intercourse within 72 hours
- those who have been raped within 72 hours

- those with known or possible condom failure within 72 hours
- those with known or suspected diaphragm/cap problems (e.g. dislodgement during intercourse) within 72 hours
- those using *coitus interruptus* within 72 hours
- those with potential combined pill failures — two or more pills missed from the first seven pills in a packet [5], or four or more pills missed midpacket [5]
- progestogen-only pill users who have missed one or more pills or taken them more than 3 hours late
- those with complete or partial expulsion of an intrauterine device (IUD) or when removal is essential midcycle
- those who attend late for a repeat Depo-Provera hormonal contraception injection

CONTRAINDICATIONS

The only WHO grade 4 contraindications for the use of POEC are established pregnancy, acute active porphyria, and active liver disease. The Yuzpe regimen is no longer available in the UK but contraindications were pregnancy, focal migraine at the time of presentation, acute active porphyria, and sickle cell crisis.

EFFICACY

Neither the Yuzpe regimen nor the POEC pill provides contraception for the remainder of the cycle, therefore it is essential to discuss a long-term method of contraception with each client. The WHO study [2] showed that each method was more effective if administered as soon as possible after unprotected intercourse (see Table 9.1). Also, both methods are more effective if intercourse is avoided until after the onset of the next period.

The study showed that 12 out of 619 women that used the Yuzpe regimen became pregnant if further intercourse was avoided whereas this figure rose to 19 out of 360 women who reported further sexual intercourse during that cycle. Of those women who used POEC, 5 out of 620 became pregnant if no further sexual activity occurred, compared to 6 out of 372 of those who had further sexual intercourse (see Table 9.2) [2].

	No sexual intercourse	Further sexual intercourse
Yuzpe regimen	1.9%	5.3%
POEC	0.8%	1.6%

Table 9.2 Percentage of women that became pregnant using the Yuzpe regimen or the progestogen-only emergency contraceptive pill with and without further sexual intercourse during the current menstrual cycle [2].

Although both the Yuzpe regimen and POEC are much less effective if initiated more than 72 hours after the initial unprotected act of coitus, late presentation is not an absolute contraindication.

The postcoital intrauterine device

Any copper-bearing coil can be used as emergency contraception. Approximately 7000 postcoital coils were fitted at family planning clinics in England in 1999 [1].

MODE OF ACTION

As a copper IUD is usually inserted after ovulation, its main mode of action is to block implantation. However, if fitted early in the cycle it may prevent fertilization. The Mirena intrauterine system is not recommended for postcoital use.

EFFICACY

The postcoital IUD has the highest efficacy of any emergency contraception method currently available. The failure rate is estimated to be around 0.1% [6].

WHO SHOULD HAVE AN EMERGENCY COPPER COIL FITTED?

A copper-bearing coil can be fitted up to 5 days after unprotected intercourse or up to 5 days after the expected date of ovulation, i.e. up to day 19 of a 28 day cycle. Therefore, it can be offered when:

- multiple acts of coitus have occurred – the first more than 72 hours earlier
- the client presents late for hormonal emergency contraception
- the most effective method is required
- the client was considering an IUD as a long-term contraception method

The greatest risk of pelvic inflammatory disease is within 20 days of IUD insertion [7]. Women should have a follow-up examination approximately 3 weeks after the fitting. The coil can be removed with the next menses or be left in place to provide ongoing contraception. GyneFIX is the only currently marketed IUD to have a license for use as a postcoital coil. The postcoital IUD has the same contraindications for use as a copper IUD (see Chapter 7).

CHLAMYDIA SCREENING

Women seeking emergency contraception have, by definition, had unprotected intercourse, therefore a sexual history should be taken and chlamydia screening should be offered. Insertion of an IUD can impair the cervical mechanisms that protect the upper genital tract from infection, therefore chlamydia screening is also recommended for all women prior to insertion of a postcoital coil. Women testing positively for chlamydia should be treated with a 7-day course of doxycycline (100 mg twice daily) or azithromycin (1 g). Contact tracing and treatment of the partners of chlamydia-positive women should be instigated.

Managing a request for emergency contraception

When managing a request for emergency contraception, the following must be documented:

- the first day of the last menstrual period (LMP)
- the length of the cycle
- the timing of all inadequately protected intercourse during the current cycle

If the date or the character of the LMP indicates that the woman could already be pregnant, a pregnancy test must be carried out before any medication is prescribed. When emergency contraception is prescribed, it is important to discuss:

- how the method works
- possible side effects, such as nausea and vomiting
- possible effects on the menstrual cycle – bleeding may occur a few days after taking hormonal emergency contraception and immediately after the fitting of an IUD. Most women will have their next period around the expected time but it may be a few days early or late [2]
- efficacy
- return for a pregnancy test if the next period is more than 7 days late
- abstinence or very careful use of a barrier method until onset of the next period if hormonal treatment is used
- the need for ongoing reliable contraception

Accessibility of emergency contraception

Levonelle has been licensed for sale as an over-the-counter medication since January 2001 in the UK, and can be purchased by women over the age of 16 years for approximately £20. It is hoped that this will make emergency contraception more accessible to women and that usage will increase. Levonelle may also be obtained free of charge at all family planning clinics and from most GPs and genitourinary medicine clinics. Some A&E departments also provide emergency contraception.

Many areas are considering 'patient group directions' for the supply of Levonelle. Patient group directions allow any healthcare professional to supply a prescription-only medication directly to a patient provided that a set of guidelines, agreed with a doctor, are followed. Levonelle could then be administered by school nurses, often on school premises, or by practice nurses running teenage 'drop-in' clinics. Again it is hoped that easier access will result in an increased uptake of emergency contraception, reducing the number of unplanned teenage pregnancies. If these options are to have any impact on unplanned pregnancies, careful use of a suitable protocol and guidance on long-term contraception will be essential.

References

1. NHS Contraceptive Services, England 1999–2000 Statistical Bulletin. Available at: http://www.doh.gov.uk/pdfs/sb0027.pdf.

2. The WHO Task Force on Postovulatory Methods of Fertility Regulation. Randomised controlled trial of levonorgestrel versus the Yuzpe regimen of combined oral contraception for emergency contraception. *Lancet* 1998;352:428–33.

3. Trussell J, Rodriguez G, Ellertson C. Updated estimates of the effectiveness of the Yuzpe regimen of emergency contraception. *Contraception* 1999;59:147–51.

4. Wilcox AJ, Dunson D, Baird DD. The timing of the 'fertile window' in the menstrual cycle: day specific estimates from a prospective study. *BMJ* 2000;321:1259–62.

5. Guidance on emergency contraception; recommendations for clinical practice. Faculty of Family Planning and Reproductive Healthcare. Royal College of Obstetricians and Gynaecologists (RCOG), April 2000.

6. Van Look PF, Stewart F. Emergency contraception. In: *Contraceptive technology*. 17th revised edition. Hatcher RA, Trussell J, Stewart F, editors. New York: Irvington Publishers, 1998.

7. Farley TM, Rosenberg MJ, Rowe PJ. Intrauterine devices and pelvic inflammatory disease: an international perspective. *Lancet* 1992;339:785–8.

chapter 10

Sex, teenagers, and health professionals

Marian Everett

In 1992, a UK government white paper recognized the importance of teenage sexual health and that action was required to reduce the unacceptably high levels of teenage pregnancy and sexually transmitted infections (STIs). One of the targets of 'The Health of The Nation' was to halve the conception rate in 13–15 year olds to 4.8 per 1000, by the year 2000 [1].

This white paper recognized the need to accept teenage sexuality and that appropriate sex education should be provided through schools, the media, and parents prior to the onset of sexual activity. It was also recommended that contraceptive services should be easy to access, user-friendly, confidential, and non-judgmental. These targets were not met and the current Sexual Health Strategy aims to halve the number of pregnancies in under 18 year olds by the year 2010.

To give an idea of the extent of the problem, a study by the Social Exclusion Unit [2] reported that, every year in England, there are:

- 90 000 conceptions in teenagers
- 7700 conceptions in girls under 16 years old
- 2000 conceptions in girls under 14 years old
- 56 000 live births in teenagers

The problem affects every part of the UK. It is worse in poorer areas, with particularly high rates of pregnancy occurring in the most vulnerable groups of young people. These vulnerable groups are: teenage girls in local authority housing; children in care; children of teenage mothers; young girls who are excluded from school; teenagers aged 16 and 17 who are not in education, training, or work; and young people who have been sexually abused.

Teenagers – the facts

- half of the teenagers who are sexually active use no contraception the first time they have sex

- of those who become pregnant, half of the under 16 year olds and a third of 16 and 17 year olds opt for abortion – 15 000 young people under the age of 18 have an abortion every year
- the majority (90%) of teenage mothers are not married and there is a high chance that their relationship will break down
- teenage parents are more likely than their peers to live in poverty, to be unemployed, and to drop out of education
- the death rate for babies of teenage mothers is higher than for babies of older mothers, and they are more likely to have low birth weights

Why are teenage pregnancy rates so high in the UK?

Other countries reduced their teenage pregnancy rates in the 1980s and 1990s. What happened to the UK?

IGNORANCE
Teenagers lack accurate knowledge about contraception. Only about half of under 16 year olds, and two thirds of 16–19 year olds, use contraception when they first become sexually active, compared with 80% in the Netherlands. The reality of bringing up a child alone and on a low income is not discussed. Teenagers do not know how easy it is to get pregnant and how hard it is to be a parent.

MIXED MESSAGES
The adult world tells young people that sexual activity is normal, through advertising, television programs, magazines, and films. However, educational institutions and parents find sex a difficult and embarrassing subject. Sex education starts too late, and many teenagers are already sexually active before they receive contraceptive advice at school. There is little point in starting sex education at the age of 15 if teenagers are sexually active at 13 years old.

LOW EXPECTATIONS
Worldwide teenage pregnancy is more common in young people with low education and career expectations. There are many teenagers in the UK who can see no prospect of getting a job and, therefore, no reason to continue in education. They have little incentive not to become pregnant.

Government plans to address the issue

In an attempt to achieve its 2010 target, the government has appointed teenage pregnancy coordinators to address local needs. A national multimedia campaign is planned, using adverts in teen magazines and on local radio stations, giving the following messages:

- you choose when to have sex
- if you are sexually active, use contraception
- whatever your age, you can get free confidential advice about contraception

New guidance has been published around sex and relationships for use in schools [3]. All schools must have a sex and relationship education policy based around a lifelong learning process addressing the physical, moral, and emotional development of young people. The Department of Education and Employment recommends that this policy should be taught via the Physical Health and Social Education and citizenship frameworks, and its development should involve parents, young people, and teachers [3].

A review of studies on the effects of sex education in schools in 1993 reported that sex education does not promote earlier or increased sexual activity in young people [4]. All the data from 19 studies appeared to show that sex education leads to safer sex practices.

Holland has the lowest rate of teenage pregnancy in the world. One of the reasons for its success has been sex education in schools. Emotional and relationship issues are taught from a young age enabling discussion and forward planning between partners, a later age of first intercourse, more effective contraceptive use, and lower levels of subsequent regret about a first sexual experience. Not everyone agrees with this approach [5], but a policy of advising teenagers not to have sex does not work and may deter teenagers from accessing the sexual health services that are available to them.

Parents have the right to withdraw their children from all or part of the sex and relationship education provided at school, except for those parts included in the National Curriculum (see Figure 10.1) [3].

What do teenagers want from a sexual health service?

In 1998, the Brook Advisory Center commissioned a report: 'What young people want from sexual health services' [6]. Young people formed focus groups to identify the characteristics of their ideal service. Conclusions revealed that young people wanted a sexual health service that was confidential and easy to access with minimum fear

NATIONAL CURRICULUM SCIENCE

Key Stage 1

1. b) that animals including humans, move, feed, grow, use their senses and reproduce.

2. a) to recognise and compare the main external parts of the bodies of humans

   f) that humans and animals can produce offspring and these grow into adults

4 a) to recognise similarities and differences between themselves and others and treat others with sensitivity

Key Stage 2

1. a) that the life processes common to humans and other animals include nutrition, growth and reproduction

2. f) about the main stages of the human life cycle

Key Stage 3

1. d) that fertilisation in humans... is the fusion of a male and a female cell

2. f) about the physical and emotional changes that take place during adolescence

   g) about the human reproductive system, including the menstrual cycle and fertilisation

   h) how the foetus develops in the uterus

   n) how the growth and reproduction of bacteria and the replication of viruses can affect health

Key Stage 4

2. f) the way in which hormonal control occurs, including the effects of sex hormones

   g) some medical uses of hormones, including the control and promotion of fertility

   l) the defence mechanisms of the body

3. d) how sex is determined in humans

Figure 10.1 Sex and Relationship Education Guidance included in the National Curriculum (UK) [3].

and embarrassment. The ideal clinic would be located on a side street in the town center, would have frequent opening times, modern premises, and should be able to be used in a 'walk in' capacity. The clinic should be staffed by friendly, respectful, non-judgmental staff who are well informed on gay and lesbian issues, making no assumptions about heterosexuality.

In November 2000, the Teenage Pregnancy Unit at the Department of Health issued best practice advice on the provision of effective contraceptive and advisory services to young people [7]. This advisory document suggested that young people should be involved locally in planning and evaluating services, with particular input into the location and opening times of clinics, publicity, and the generation of user-friendly literature. Confidentiality is of paramount importance to young people and all services should have an explicit confidentiality policy, which should be displayed prominently.

Contraception without parental consent

Following the 1985 House of Lords ruling in the case of *Gillick vs. West Norfolk and Wisbech Area Health Authority* [8], doctors can give contraceptive advice and treatment to young people under the age of 16 years without parental consent, provided the conditions as ruled by the law are fulfilled. These conditions are outlined in the Frazer guidelines, which are provided below:

- the young person understands the advice and has sufficient maturity to understand what is involved
- the young person can not be persuaded to inform the parents and will not allow the doctor to do so
- the young person is likely to begin or continue to have sexual intercourse with or without contraception
- without contraception the young person's physical or mental health will suffer
- it is in the young person's best interests to give advice or treatment or both, with or without parental consent

The phrase 'Gillick competency' is often used when dealing with young adolescents. Competency is understood in terms of the patient's ability to understand the choices, and the consequences of these choices, including the nature, purpose, and possible risk of any treatment (or non-treatment). Parental consent to treatment is not necessary [9]. It is desirable that young people have parental support and this should be discussed during the consultation. Often the young person does not wish to involve the parents, and the doctor must respect this decision in the vast majority of cases.

Two other documents have helped to guide sexual health services for under 16 year olds. The first report, 'The 1989 Children Act', states that children under the age of 16 years may be able to give or refuse consent depending on their capacity to understand the nature of the treatment [10]. Whether or not the young person understands is a decision for the doctor. The second document, 'Confidentiality and People Under 16 Years', is another useful guide for healthcare professionals [9]. This states that: "The duty of confidentiality owed to a person under 16 is as great as that owed to any other person. Regardless of whether or not the requested treatment is given, the confidentiality of the consultation should be respected unless there are convincing reasons to the contrary."

No patient, adult or minor, has a right to absolute confidentiality in all circumstances. If the doctor believes that the client is suffering abuse, or if other vulnerable people are at risk, then it may be necessary to breach confidentiality. However, it is essential to inform the client that a disclosure must be made, even if the client continues to withhold consent.

Consent for abortion

If the doctor is satisfied that a girl under the age of 16 years old understands the nature of the procedure, the possible complications, the issues invoked, and she refuses to involve her parents, then the Frazer guidelines may be used. If the doctor believes it to be in the girl's best interests to go ahead with an abortion then the procedure may be carried out.

Teenage sexual health services

Young people only tend to access sexual health services in a crisis situation. Often this will be to obtain emergency contraception or have a pregnancy test, i.e. after unprotected intercourse. Attendance is spasmodic as the teenager lurches from one crisis to another. Long-term contraception must be discussed and, if possible, provided during these intermittent attendances. However, even if successfully provided, long-term contraception is often abandoned as young people practice serial monogamy, moving from one short-term relationship to another, with the risks of unintended pregnancy or contracting an STI. Contraception is usually the first casualty of a breakdown in a relationship – young women will stop taking the pill midpacket and, if a reconciliation occurs, unprotected intercourse and its consequences result.

Any young person attending sexual health services for the first time is likely to be nervous, embarrassed, and anxious. The consultation must not be rushed and it is essential that confidentiality is assured. All methods of contraception should be briefly mentioned and the preferred method discussed in detail. There is no need to do a pelvic or breast examination in any woman prior to commencing contraception (unless there are strong clinical indications to do so) [11]. The consultation is an ideal opportunity to talk about relationships and feelings, and promote safer sex. The attitude of the health professionals is vital and must be non-judgmental, sympathetic, and supportive.

Children deserve an open relationship with teachers and sex education appropriate to their age all the way through school. Parents need to be encouraged to talk to their children, and one of the roles of the teenage pregnancy coordinator will be to involve parents and carers in sex education. Services must be appropriate to the needs of young people and their views should be taken into account when seeking to address the problem of teenage pregnancy in the UK.

References

1. The Health of the Nation: a strategy for health in England. London: HMSO, 1992.

2. Teenage pregnancy – a report by the Social Exclusion Unit, June 1999.

3. Sex and Relationship Education Guidance. Ref. DfEE 0116/2000, DfEE, July 2000

4. Baldo M, Aggleton P. Does sex education lead to earlier or increased sexual activity in youth? IXth International Conference on AIDS. Berlin, Abstract D02-3444, 1993.

5. Stammers T, Ingham R. For and against: doctors should advise adolescents to abstain from sex. *BMJ* 2000;321:1520–2.

6. Someone with a smile would be your best bet. What young people want from a sexual health service? London: The Brook Advisory Centre, March 1988.

7. Best practice advice on the provision of effective contraception and advice services for young people. Teenage pregnancy unit, Department of Health, 2000.

8. *Gillick vs. West Norfolk and Wisbech Area Health Authority*, 3 All ER 402 HL (1985).

9. Confidentiality and people under 16. Guidance issued jointly by the BMA, GMSC, HEA, Brook Advisory Centres, FPA and RCG, 1994.

10. Working together under the children act 1989. London: HMSO, 1991.

11. Faculty of Family Planning and Reproductive Health Care. Royal College of Obstetricians and Gynaecologists. First prescription of combined oral contraception: recommendations for clinical practice. *Br J Fam Plann* 2000;26:27–38.

chapter 11

Unplanned pregnancy

Marian Everett

No woman expects that she will ever conceive an unwanted child, or need to have an abortion. An unplanned pregnancy is not necessarily unwanted, but many planned pregnancies can become unwanted due to changing circumstances.

Why is abortion necessary?

Abortion is necessary for complete fertility control for a number of reasons:

- there is an imbalance between sexuality and rationality
- the urge to have sex is difficult to balance with 'safe sex'
- successful use of contraception requires communication between partners
- contraception is not very effective, even when used properly

For example, the failure rate of the combined oral contraceptive pill is quoted as 0.1% with perfect use, but can be as high as 5% with typical use [1]. Therefore, if 3 million women are taking the pill, even with perfect use, there will be 3000 pregnancies per year. The failure rate of condoms can be as high as 15%, leading to many thousands of unplanned pregnancies.

An unwanted pregnancy can threaten the mental, physical, and social well-being of the mother. A woman's acceptance of an unintended pregnancy depends on how she perceives her capacity to be a parent. Other factors, such as her role in society, and her socio-economic and educational status, may also affect her decision.

The 1967 Abortion Act

The 1967 Abortion Act (amended by the 1990 Human Fertilization and Embryology Act) allows the termination of pregnancy (TOP) if, in the opinion of two doctors, it threatens the mental or physical health of the woman or of her existing children.

Most doctors accept the World Health Organization (WHO) definition of health as "a state of physical and mental well-being and not just an absence of disease." The act encourages doctors, when making their decision, to take into account the woman's actual or foreseeable circumstances. The act has eliminated illegal abortions in England by allowing safe abortion to be performed by qualified doctors under regulated circumstances.

The 1967 Abortion Act is applicable throughout the UK, with the exception of Northern Ireland. Approximately 2000 women travel to England each year from Northern Ireland to have an abortion.

Confirming a pregnancy

When a woman suspects she may be pregnant, she will usually seek confirmation by carrying out a pregnancy test. She may choose to buy a kit and do a home test. She may take a sample to her general practitioner (GP), a family planning clinic, a chemist's shop, or a genitourinary medicine (GUM) clinic. Most women are able to assess the advantages and disadvantages of continuing with the pregnancy and have made a decision before consulting a doctor. All women need a sympathetic, non-judgmental doctor when they do seek help.

At this stage, the options available to the woman are to continue with the pregnancy and bring up the child, or have the baby adopted, or to terminate the pregnancy. The doctor can guide the woman towards social services if information is required about financial support or housing. For pregnant teenagers, many areas have established 'Sure Start Plus' which provides one-to-one information about making the decision to carry on with the pregnancy or have an abortion. Teenage parents also receive an integrated support package to get them back into education, training, or employment.

Some hospitals have separate antenatal clinics and support groups for teenagers, run by midwives. These organizations can also help with breaking the news of pregnancy to the teenage girl's parents or carers.

Reasons for abortion

The majority of abortions (97%) are carried out because the pregnancy threatens the mental health of the mother or her existing children. Approximately 1.5% of abortions are carried out because of danger to the physical health of the mother, and 1% because the fetus is likely to be seriously abnormal. Abortions to protect the life of the pregnant woman form a very small proportion of the total.

Abortion for 'social reasons' must be carried out before 24 weeks' gestation, but is legal at any time during the pregnancy if the woman's life is at risk or there is a risk of serious fetal abnormality. Most abortions (90%) are carried out before 13 weeks' gestation, with 98% being carried out before 20 weeks' gestation. In the UK, only about 100 occur annually after 24 weeks [2].

The majority of women suspecting an unwanted pregnancy will see their GP for help and advice. Some women may feel that a request for abortion will result in the loss of their doctor's respect. Often, women will be worried that their GP may have conscientious objections to abortion, or fear an unsympathetic or judgmental response. Some women, especially young adolescents, will be concerned about confidentiality issues. Many are ambivalent about the decision and will welcome nondirective counseling.

If the woman is sure about her decision to terminate the pregnancy, the GP may feel able to make the referral and sign the first part of certificate A (see Figure 11.1) [3]. If not, the GP must help the woman to consult a colleague who will make the referral. If this does not occur, then the GP is in breach of the terms and conditions of his or her service. A woman may choose to seek advice from a doctor other than her GP. This is also true when she is seeking maternity or contraceptive services.

Many women will attend family planning or GUM clinics for direct referral to abortion services. About 30% of women go straight to a private organization [4]. Some areas have direct access to National Health Service (NHS) abortion facilities and women can self-refer directly to the abortion provider.

Abortion options available

When a decision to terminate has been made, the options available will depend upon the length of gestation and where the woman lives (not all areas will have a full range of abortion options available on the NHS).

EARLY MEDICAL ABORTION

Early medical abortion can be carried out up to day 63 of gestation. The procedure is carried out in two stages. The first stage is the oral administration of 200 mg of mifepristone. The second stage is carried out 36–48 hours later when 1 mg of gemeprost, or 800 μg of misoprostol (unlicensed use), are inserted into the vagina. The cervix dilates and the uterus contracts to expel the products, usually within 3 hours of the insertion of the prostaglandin (gemeprost/misoprostol). The efficacy

---

IN CONFIDENCE

CERTIFICATE A

ABORTION ACT 1967

Not to be destroyed within three years of the date of operation

**Certificate to be completed before an abortion is
performed under Section 1(1) of the Act**

I, ...
(Name and qualifications of practitioner in block capitals)

of ....

....
(Full address of practitioner)

Have/have not* seen/and examined* the pregnant woman to whom this certificate relates at

....

....
(full address of place at which patient was seen or examined)

on ....

and I ....
(Name and qualifications of practitioner in block capitals)

of ....

....
(Full address of practitioner)

Have/have not* seen/and examined* the pregnant woman to whom this certificate relates at

....

....
(Full address of place at which patient was seen or examined)

on ....

We hereby certify that we are of the opinion, formed in good faith, that in the case

of ....
(Full name of pregnant woman in block capitals)

of ....

....
(Usual place of residence of pregnant woman in block capitals)

(Ring appro-priate letter(s))

A   the continuance of the pregnancy would involve risk to the life of the pregnant woman greater than if the pregnancy were terminated;

B   the termination is necessary to prevent grave permanent injury to the physical or mental health of the pregnant woman;

C   the pregnancy has NOT exceeded its 24th week and that the continuance of the pregnancy would involve risk, greater than if the pregnancy were terminated, of injury to the physical or mental health of the pregnant woman;

D   the pregnancy has NOT exceeded its 24th week and that the continuance of the pregnancy would involve risk, greater than if the pregnancy were terminated, of injury to the physical or mental health of any existing child(ren) of the family of the pregnant woman;

E   there is a substantial risk that if the child were born it would suffer from such physical or mental abnormalities as to be seriously handicapped.

This certificate of opinion is given before the commencement of the treatment for the termination of pregnancy to which it refers and relates to the circumstances of the pregnant woman's individual case.

Signed ....   **Date** ....

Signed ....   **Date** ....

* Delete as appropriate   Printed in the U.K. for H.M.S.O. 5/'91 Dd. DH001306 C10000 38806 G3994   Form HSA1 (revised 1991)

Figure 11.1 Certificate A of the Abortion Act 1967 [3].

of early medical abortion is similar to surgical abortion; complete abortion occurs in 97–98% of women [5]. Further surgical evacuation will be required by 2%–3% to remove retained products of conception and a further 1% will require intervention because of an ongoing pregnancy.

SUCTION TERMINATION

This method can be used between weeks 7–14 of gestation. It is usually carried out under general anesthetic as a day-case procedure. Cervical priming with gemeprost, misoprostol, or mifepristone is recommended for gestations over 10 weeks or in women under 18 years old [6]. A bimanual examination is carried out, the cervix is dilated appropriate to the gestation, and a suction catheter is introduced into the uterine cavity. The uterus is emptied using gentle suction and the cavity is checked with sponge holders and a curette.

MANUAL VACUUM ASPIRATION

This method can be used between 5–12 weeks' gestation. The cervix is not dilated and the uterine contents are removed with a 6 mm Karman catheter and a hand-held syringe. The procedure is performed under local anesthetic or even 'vocal local' – the presence of a reassuring nurse is often sufficient [7].

MEDICAL ABORTION OVER 13 WEEKS

Various regimes are used:

- mifepristone, 600 mg orally, followed 36–48 hours later by gemeprost, 1 mg vaginally, repeated every 3 hours, to a maximum of five pessaries (licensed)
- mifepristone, 200 mg orally, followed 36–48 hours later by misoprostol, 800 μg vaginally and 400 μg orally every 3 hours, to a maximum of four doses (unlicensed)

With these methods, surgical evacuation is not usually necessary.

DILATION AND EVACUATION

This method may be used for abortions of 15 weeks' gestation and above. The cervix is primed as for a surgical abortion (with gemeprost, misoprostol, or mifepristone) and the uterus is emptied using special instruments. The gynecologist must have an adequate caseload to keep up his or her skills [6].

ABORTION COMPLICATIONS

- hemorrhage (1.5 per 1000 abortions). The rate is lower for early abortions
- uterine perforation (1 to 4 per 1000 surgical abortions). Laparoscopy is the investigation of choice if a perforation is suspected

- failed abortion/ongoing pregnancy. This is more likely with vacuum aspiration under 7 weeks' gestation or with early medical abortion
- infection (10% of abortions). The risk can be minimized by screening and/or treating prophylactically with antibiotics. The prevalence of chlamydia is quoted as 5%–12% in women having TOPs in the UK [8]
- psychological problems – early distress is common. Only a small minority of women have long-term psychological problems, including psychosexual problems
- there is no proven association between induced abortion and subsequent infertility [6]

The assessment clinic

The assessment clinic should be staffed by health professionals who are sympathetic to women seeking abortion. Ideally, this clinic should be separate from gynecology services and should definitely be separate from maternity services. Facilities for counseling and access to social services should be available.

THE PRE-ABORTION ASSESSMENT

When making a pre-abortion assessment, a patient history, including obstetric and gynecological histories, should be taken. A note should be made of any medication that is currently being prescribed. A pelvic examination should be performed (this may include cervical cytology if appropriate), as well as an ultrasound scan when the gestation is in doubt or an extrauterine pregnancy is suspected [6]. Hemoglobin levels and the ABO and Rhesus status should be assessed. Many units offer screening for sexually transmitted infections (STIs), especially chlamydia [8]. The need for ongoing contraception must be discussed and prescribed if appropriate. An intrauterine device or contraceptive implant can be inserted at the end of a surgical procedure. Depo-Provera, the combined pill, the progestogen only pill, or Implanon can be started on the same day as a medical or surgical abortion.

Many units offer prophylactic antibiotics, e.g. a 7-day treatment with doxycycline, 100 mg twice daily, and metronidazole, 1 g rectally at the time of surgical procedure. This should be discussed and consent should be obtained for rectal administration prior to the procedure being carried out. If swabs for STIs are taken, it is essential that contact details are available so that the results can be communicated to the woman later. In the event of a positive result, contact tracing and treatment of the partner(s) is mandatory, and many units have good arrangements in place with their local GUM clinic [8].

How can abortion services be improved?

- all women requesting an abortion should be offered an assessment within 5 days, and certainly within 2 weeks, of referral [6]
- the abortion should ideally be carried out within 7 days, and certainly within 2 weeks, of the assessment
- no women should wait more than 3 weeks between referral and abortion [6]
- health authorities should meet the local need for legal abortion – in Scotland 98.5% of abortions are funded by the NHS; in Solihull the figure is only 46% [9]
- GP practice leaflets should indicate whether they are prepared to refer women for legal abortions
- early abortion could be provided in centers other than NHS hospitals, e.g. GP surgeries and family planning clinics

All women should have access to safe abortion, provided by sympathetic, non-judgmental healthcare professionals, who are knowledgeable about the options available, the potential complications, the risks of STIs, and the need for contraception afterwards.

References

1. Trussell J. Contraceptive failure rates 1994. In: Hatcher RA, Trussell J, Stewart F et al, editors. *Contraceptive Technology*. 17th revised edition. New York: Irvington Publishers, 1998:637–87.

2. Office for National Statistics. 1996 Abortion Statistics: England and Wales, series AB no. 23. London: The Stationery Office, 1997.

3. Certificate A. Abortion Act 1967. Form HSA1 (revised 1991). London: HMSO.

4. Birth Control Trust. Abortion Provision in Britain - How services are provided and how they could be improved (1997) London: Birth Control Trust.

5. Cameron ST, Glaisier AF, Logan J et al. Impact of the introduction of new medical methods on therapeutic abortions at the Royal Infirmary of Edinburgh. *Br J Obstet Gynaecol* 1996;103:1222–9.

6. Royal College of Obstetrics and Gynaecology. The care of women requesting induced abortion. Guideline no. 7. March, 2000. London: RCOG Press.

7. Boorer C, Murty J. Experience of termination of pregnancy in a stand-alone clinic situation. *J Fam Plann Reprod Health Care* 2001;27:97–8.

8. Groom TM, Stewart P, Kruger H et al. The value of a screen and treat policy for *Chlamydia trachomatis* in women attending for termination of pregnancy. *J Fam Plann Reprod Health Care* 2001;27:69–72.

9. The Abortion Law Reform Association (ALRA): Campaign for Choice. NHS Abortion Provision. Available from: URL: http://www.alra.org.uk/nhs.html.

Abbreviations

A&E	accident and emergency
AIDS	acquired immunodeficiency syndrome
BTB	breakthrough bleeding
BV	bacterial vaginosis
CMO	Chief Medical Officer
COC	combined oral contraception
CS	Cesarean section
DNA	deoxyribonucleic acid
EIA	enzyme immunoassay
ESR	erythrocyte sedimentation rate
GBS	group B streptococcus
GP	general practitioner
GUM	genitourinary medicine
hCG	human chorionic gonadotropin
HIV	human immunodeficiency virus
HPV	human papillomavirus
HSV	herpes simplex virus
IM	intramuscular
IUD	intrauterine device
IUS	intrauterine system
IV	intravenous
LGTI	lower genital tract infection
LH	luteinizing hormone
LMP	last menstrual period
OR	odds ratio
Pap	Papanicolaou
PCR	polymerase chain reaction
PID	pelvic inflammatory disease
POEC	progestogen-only emergency contraceptive
POP	progesterone only pill
STI	sexually transmitted infection
TOP	termination of pregnancy
WHO	World Health Organization

Index

in pregnancy 66–67
aqueous cream 30

B
bacterial vaginosis (BV) 33–37
   intermenstrual bleeding 53
   pregnancy 68
Bartholin's gland abscess 49–50
birthrate
   teenage 109, 110
      by European countries 7
bleeding
   breakthrough 89–90
   intermenstrual 53
   postcoital 53
bone density, Depo-Provera 96
breakthrough bleeding 89–90

C
candida infections 37–40
   recurrence 39–40
cervical specimen 13–15
Cesarean section
   herpes infection 66–67
   HIV infection 69–70
chlamydial infections 43–47
   complications 47
   epidemiology 1, 3
     COC use 5
   neonates 64
   pregnancy 63–64
     ectopic/tubal 58–59, 63–64
   recurrence 46
   see also pelvic inflammatory disease
coitus interruptus 78
combined oral contraception (COC) 85–91

E

F

G

urethral specimen 13–15
urethritis 30–32

V
vaginal discharge 33–50
vaginosis *see* bacterial vaginosis
vulval lesions
    dermatoses 30
    irritation 29–30
    lumps 17–22
    ulcers 22–28
vulvitis 30–32

W
weight gain 90–91

Y
Yuzpe regimen, emergency contraception 103–106

Coventry University